the perfect servant ...nope

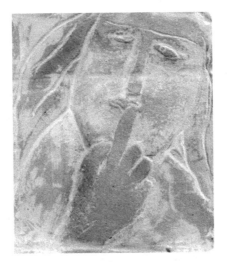

shhhh... don't tell

a caregiver's hat from hell

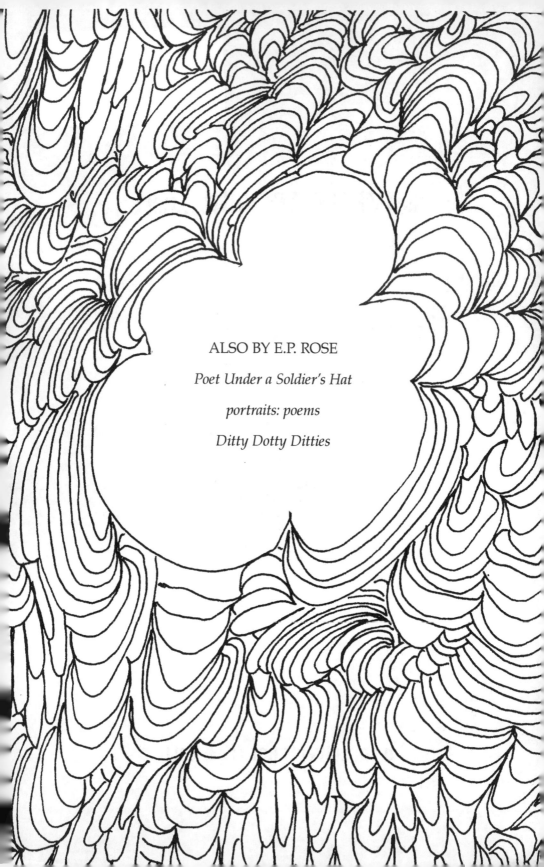

ALSO BY E.P. ROSE

Poet Under a Soldier's Hat

portraits: poems

Ditty Dotty Ditties

e.p. rose

E. P. Rose

the perfect servant ...nope

a caregiver's hat from hell

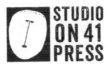

STUDIO
ON 41
PRESS

First Edition

Studio on 41 Press
Galisteo, New Mexico
www.galisteoliz.com

Book design: Donna Brownell
Illustrations: David Burk

Printed in the U.S.A.

ISBN: 978-0-9861188-6-9

for all of us not so perfect servants, helping those who need us.

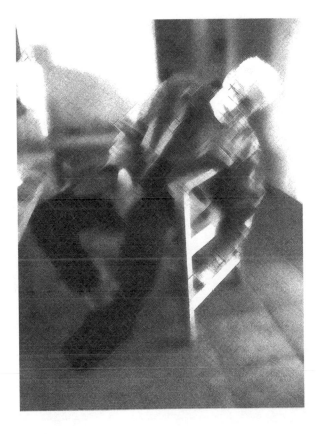

preface
why blog?

"OOO," I thought, during a lecture on blogging. "Write a blog. There's something I'd like to do," and that said, signed up for a six-session course.

A theme came easily. Caregiving. The daily hell of it. For who spoke for us?

Me-an impulsive *up-and-at-it* antsy kind of being with little patience for rules, timetables and going slow, poor David, my long-suffering husband, Parkinson's couldn't have inflicted on him a worse nursemaid.

Can you imagine? I actually retched the first time I changed my first newborn's dirty nappy. Laughable considering the horrors I take in my stride today.

Just the two of us at home alone, trapped, desperate, I became a foul companion.

Dull-haired, a woman's face in the mirror searched mine with a scary wildness in her eyes I didn't like or want to be around.

The Perfect Servant I was not, and so my blog was born.

Though quite against my British nature, in it I would voice all those no-no thoughts and emotional swings I and other caregivers are not supposed to think, feel, nor ever say aloud.

My thought...better to vent depressing woes in a blog rather than moan on endlessly and risk losing my friends.

Surprisingly the act of scribing words on paper, well the computer, was as though I was talking to a person. Sympathetic. One willing to accept my raging, and help me clarify my course of action.

Recording my caregiving journey and our dilemma has changed me for sure.

Mostly my anger has faded. David and I have fun again. Acceptance...my new attitude is the key.

The difference in tone between my first and last blog is undeniable proof. From the letters I've received, seems other caregivers have found help too.

Best of all, by blogging I've discovered the simple truth of how much love David and I have for eachother. I so want him to stay forever.

Thank goodness for David's sweet and lovely nature—the glue that keeps me from falling apart.

Spring is upon us here in New Mexico. This Land of Enchantment is in bloom. David has even sprouted a little extra hair.

How's that for something to celebrate? Plus, we've a big party coming up in June. A sort of wake with friends and family while we're still alive.

"You could call it an *awake*," giggled a friend.

"Sounds like fun reunion. I'd like to be there," David insisted.

And so, fate-willing, he... we will.

acknowledgements

A big thank you to my brave and patient husband, David, and every victim of Parkinson's and other disabilities—both sufferers and caregivers, and to the readers of my blog for being there, and especially to my book designer, Donna Brownell, without whose untiring help and enthusiasm this book could never have materialized

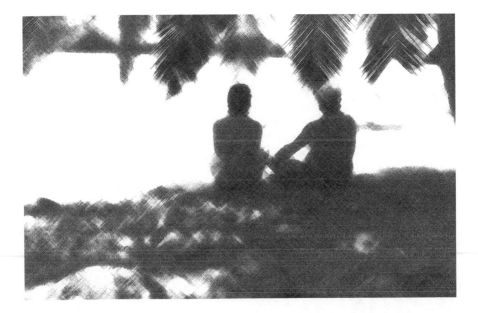

November 4, 2016

1. wearinG a hat from heLL

I have never written a blog. Don't quite know what a blog is. The one blog I have read was part of a novel. As far as I can tell blogs are rants. Mental diarrhea spilled on a page for strangers. So, fellow caregivers wearing a hat from hell, do you talk of ending it all? Use the no-no word — *death?*

Ooops. Aren't I supposed to love my role, the God-given opportunity of service, the privileged chance to score a heaven-entry ticket like the pre-check and global card we flash to airport security?

Admit it people, you are persona *non-fff-ing-grata,* a feared social pariah now your partner, or whoever you're caring for, is disabled. At least I am. And, if I'm honest, I wouldn't choose us to take up space at a dinner table for six or eight—dead-weights with *need*s who don't fan witty dinner conversation.

So-called friends shy from you and your spouse at social gatherings. If they do stop to say hello, ask, "How you doing?" They move along without waiting for your reply.

"Better make the rounds," they murmur.

"Everything good?" An acquaintance purred as she passed.

Her eyes popped when I slammed back, "No. Hardly." I knew she knew of my husband's crumbling beneath the weight of Parkinson's — my crumbling too.

"We're crawling back from death," I spat. "The emergency room docs gave him a couple of hours to live."

I'm tired of making *nice-nice-everything's-fine* bullshit noises, tired of keeping people comfortable. I want authentic. A kindly ear to receive our story.

You might wonder why I was there... socializing, I mean. You might say I had no business going. I wonder why too, pretending it was fun to sip a glass of red while burbling inconsequential rubbish about the damn cottontails having eaten the new tomato plants.

"... and despite the fact their leaves are poisonous... " the woman paused, smiling.

So bunnies why didn't you roll about and die if the plant was deadly, my thoughts growled, and immediately my mind flew back to the husband I'd left at home.

"Be gone no more than half an hour," lipstick dragged across my lips, I kissed my dozing beloved's lips and fled. I craved air... a few minutes flight with my wings unfurled.

Does that make me an abuser leaving him unattended? Because I do. Sometimes two. Even three hours. Propped upright into his chair, a spill-proof drink beside him, the TV switched to a favorite channel, the phone he can hear but isn't able to dial within reach, I dangle the car keys hesitating.

"I'll be fine," he encourages. "Go. I'm OK. Go."

Three hours tops is OK I rationalize. If he fell, though it wouldn't be jolly lying unable to move that long, it wouldn't be fatal.

November 12.2016

2. back story before the tidal wave david's life sentence means life

To better get what the hell it is I'm sounding off about, I'll set the scene from fifteen year's ago before the Parkinsonian sea engulfed us, before my husband declared himself trapped alive inside a sinking wreck.

I glanced up.

Sitting in our living room, the fireplace spluttering piñon sparks, I moved the fireguard against the adobe orifice and settled back.

Newsnight, a program my husband loved, glued him to the screen. Words tossed tired, leaving the great big world unchanged. Not ours, though. Ours morphed that night, the night I noticed…

My husband David's cheeks smooth as the TV screen, the corner of his lips devoid of curl, his eyes saucer round, nodding at the key points being argued, I assumed he was taking it all in.

The interviewer on *Newsnight* leaned forward, bushy eyebrows pulled close and down, mantling personal thoughts. A smile disrupted the furrowed lines marking his cheeks. He pushed his lips forward. It was easy to see he was engaged. But my husband — was he engaged? His expression gave no hint. I picked up a cashew fragment from my lap, cast it with the doctor's words into the flames.

"*Swaha*," I sighed. "Here's to all we have this minute." The fire-log like our future, incinerated leaving only the present.

David looked the same as he did yesterday, the same sweet way he's looked for the years we've been together, the same physically since his ten o'clock doctor's appointment the previous morning.

Was that only thirty-six hours ago? David's face: the interviewer on the box. I looked from one to the other. Studied the contrast.

"You have what's known as a Parkinson's mask, an early symptom of the disease."

The doctor's words un-rumpled a list of symptoms… joint stiffness, tiredness, micrography, tremor, fears we'd scrunched inside. For a couple of months I noticed his voice. Its new sexy huskiness. And teased him.

Then not so long ago, speed walking our favorite circuit behind his house, he stopped, waited for me to catch up.

"My left arm won't swing," he complained. "I wonder. Could I have I had a mini stroke?"

Next day at the doctor's office, the doctor clicked his ballpoint pen. On. Off. On. Aligned the missile shape of it parallel between the two top lines of his notepad.

"You have Parkinson's disease." The clicking of his ballpoint spiked the silence.

The three syllables *PAR-KIN-SON'S* skimmed the surface of reality and sank beyond my conscious thought. The doctor's words were just sounds, nothing meaningful about them. After all, the sky still shimmered cloudless, and the smudge grazing the horizon too far distant to define. I was too shocked to ask what lay ahead.

Stepping from office to sunlight, we held hands, not talking. I closed my eyes felt the warmth of the sun.

Bloody ironic, David a doctor. All those nights slaving in the ER cranking extra dollars to live the poster retirement under a palm tree somewhere. Now just when he was free…

I didn't burst into tears then. It took a week. Walking one early morning along the arroyo behind our house, I brushed against a cactus. The cruel pain of its barbs gave me reason. Broke my reserve. I wept and wept.

If David cried, he cried when I was not about.

Caregivers, did you stiffen your spine like me on hearing your partner's diagnosis? *Pointless dissolving into a crybaby... pull yourself together, girl,* I admonished myself. *Face what needs facing and bloody well get on with it.*

I didn't admit to my feelings. I couldn't. I didn't recognize the *nothing* I felt covered emotions I was not strong enough to handle at that time. It's a British thing. Denial. Our way of coping.

"Let's take a trip. Go on an exploration."

So we hiked into the desert silence of White Sands and lay together beneath the Milky Way and swam the waters of Elephant Butte. For two and a half months we toured Sri Lanka, and clocked ourselves into a Kerala nursing home, South India, to undergo a month's Ayurvedic treatment, then took six weeks in a half-built ocean resort recovering.

It was a beautiful time, we agreed, riding waves twenty feet high in the Indian Ocean, strolling the Malabar coast hand in hand, eating vegetarian. We never looked or felt so healthy.

The future, not yet existent, nosing into the past, kept us warm and down-coated. Nesting, we called our *do-you-remember-when-we?...* stories.

But *PAR-KIN-SON'S* was there, three stones lying below the surface.

Dark lumps on the pristine sand, one, two, three... I could see them through the water. Behavioral and physical changes like his indecipherable writing, more frequent stumbles, fading memory, curving posture, loomed unavoidable.

What David felt, he kept to himself.

November 19, 2016

3. there's a mouse in the room

"Oh David, David," I whispered, clutching him one time in bed. "There's a mouse in the room. Listen."

We froze. There it came again scratch, scrabble, scratch. Faint. Persistent.

"It's me. My toes. On the sheet." He whispered tightening his arms about me.

Proof, definite proof Parkinson's had arrived. My *ah-ah* moment... And yours caregivers, your moment of realization? I lay awake, eyes open in the dark chasing sleep, and a future equally elusive.

We mentally ticked off TREMOR from *THE LIST.* A list of symptoms growing grimly longer.

I became defensively aware we were somehow different. Outside our home I caught people *looking*—a sly glance, a flicker of pity, unexpected kindness and some well... downright insensitive.

Incidents mounted up.

"Can't you keep your damn head still... " A woman seated behind him at a concert tapped his shoulder, snapping,

"He can't help it. He has Parkinson's." I snarled, spinning to face her,

I wanted to... did I... ? a nice person like me... ? really want to sock her one?

When next I turned round, she, the shoulder tapper, was gone. From shame I hoped.

That concert was our last. Films were alright, we agreed, if we could sit at the very back — fugitives under cover of darkness—we didn't feel good. It was more fun watching films at home on Netflix munching nuts and olives with a glass of wine.

Husband, wife, we found shelter in marriage.

"Better than going out," we agreed. Truth was, dealing with a tremor was stressful enough for the both of us without being stared at.

At a posh, white-carpeted, house warming of an acquaintance, mouths open, we, and some guests around us watched a spout of red wine do an *Old Faithful* leap from my husband's glass then drop back without spilling a single drop. We laughed all the way home.

In restaurants, eating out, Jackson Pollock spattered food and flying liquids, his lurching gait still had a funny side — just. Waiter's ran to help him from the table seeing him struggling to stand.

"HE'S NOT DRUNK. IT'S PARKINSON'S."

The looks we get. You can't imagine. I don't suppose people mean to be mean.

"Watch out," I want spit, "this could be you in so many years."

David was still autonomous; dressing, hiking, driving a car. He made our breakfast coffee, took out the garbage, but—my poor husband's body could never still. Tremors crowded his every moment. Sleep near impossible, medication zonked him unconscious.

If this is what's ahead for me the rest of my life, I'll do away with myself. David spoke without emotion.

How could I argue? It wasn't me suffering, me, who was drowning in a Parkinsonion sea. *Anyway, it's just talk, he doesn't really mean it,* I lied to myself brushing aside the choking panic seizing me, for how could anyone tremoring as he did, possibly live and be happy?

In his hands, books, magazines jiggled sentences to gibberish; the

Kindle constantly took him back to chapter one, or to unwanted pages; fingering correct computer keys became impossible; as for driving... when uncontrolled Mobius bands wove his wheels across the median, David gave up his keys, and with them his independence.

His tremor worsened to the point deep brain stimulation — DBS — was the last and only option. The neurosurgeon showed a video of the procedure; drilling, sawing through the patient's skull, the exposed, pulsating brain, the probing needle, the almond-sized implants being inserted... In place of the patient, I saw David, his brain. Too horrifically personal to watch, I fled wailing my agony into the grass surrounding his office unable to stop.

A medieval-looking iron frame screwed to his head held him immobile. I touched his lips to my lips with my finger, the only way to reach him. Still awake, the surgeon wheeled him away. Still conscious, in the operating theatre he endured the next thirteen hours.

"The drill's whine was the worst part as it broke through my skull headed for my brain," he whispered back in the ward. His pupils flared.

Did the solitary hours an earthquake victim spent trapped beneath the rubble creep as slowly as those endless hours of David's, immobile, awake, listening? As slowly as those thirteen hours I cowered alone waiting, waiting?

How I envied the overly jolly group in the room across from me spilling jokes and noisy chitchat to divert an anxious husband from thoughts of his wife — the surgeon's slicing.

Why, oh why hadn't I thought to ask a friend to be with me, keep my mind from running images I couldn't shake — blood-soaked saw-teeth, exposed pulsing brain, the burning smell of bone, David on the table? His face... I covered mine overcome, desolate.

Two gauze squares covered the wire terminals to the implants in his brain. "Devil horns," we joked driving home next day. A month later a battery was sewn into his chest and switched on.

"Look. Miracle-man. I'm back," he laughed, holding out both hands. "Bionic." His hands steady. Statue-still.

I took them and kissed his fingers.

Our lives clawed back a notch. Back to the way things had been BEFORE. We pushed Parkinson's away. Little symptoms stayed ignored… balance, worsening vision, we negotiated each new obstacle unaware we were caught in the disease's relentless current. In denial, of course. I see that now.

"Another man-quake," we joked, as I slapped Spackle into the living room wall where his elbow had punched a massive hole. Inside we were no longer laughing.

PAR-KIN-SON'S. Scratch-scrabble-scratch. A constant reminder.

> I, too am a caregiver and am very tired. I feel alone and am slowly blocking out those around me. Every day tends to feel the same. I crawl through the motions. I look forward to reading more and hope you are feeling some sense of peace, or something. I am not sure what.. -PJC

November 26, 2016

4. Shapeshifting...
husband to patient wife to caregiver

I don't recall when Parkinson's shape-shifted husband to patient, wife to caregiver. Was it the day he held up his underpants, asked, *What do I do with these?...* The day I re-taught him how to stand from sitting, use the TV remote, or the day I first wiped dignity from his backside and flushed it away?

In the mirror two heads held my gaze. I peered closer. In one face I saw me, his *Liz-darling*. The other, a crone I didn't know.

"Can't hear a word. Speak up," crone shouts craning to hear his whisper. "Use your voice... *aaah, ooo.*"

Crone models an intonation exercise.

"Hey, David your mouth," she insists tapping her chin, a reminder to close his.

"Sit up," I hear her mutter when he keels sideways in his chair... "Stand straight... Use your fork... Open your eyes... "

The orders familiar, we all know how they go. Momma-dictator ordering not a child, but a grown man, my David whom I vowed to honor and obey, to love for the rest of our lives?

I cower beneath the verbiage — the same words with which I tamed my children sixty-plus years ago, when... a single mother with a nursing baby and deaf toddler whose frustrated screeches stripped my brain.

I owned a piano then, banged Rachmaninoff's Funeral March from its ivory piano keys, sedated myself with Valium and a glass of red-too-many. Bad times. No dark night I want to visit again.

My piano long gone, art studio devoid of clay, the New Mexican soil too hard to dig, activity-till-exhaustion is what sedates — and our strict one cocktail happy hour, the hour we socialize. Well that's the idea.

"It'six. What will it be tonight, my love? G'n'T? Tequila?"

The newscaster interrupts, babbles on. No matter.

"Cheers." Our glasses salute.

Next minute his glass tilts, drenches his shirt, pants, the chair.

"Not again. How many times... ? I've told you, put your glass down on the table between sips... " My *yack-yack* strikes up again.

I flip-down the footrest, drag from my chair, stomp off for a mop, wipe him down, *sorry darling, it's not you I'm shouting at,*

"I JUST WANT ONE MOMENT'S PEACE."

Sign me up for a school for caregivers.

Hey bloggers, how come one doesn't exist?

Are you, like I am, in desperate need of tuition on conflict resolution, the delicate balance between gentle helper: versus bully, custodian: wife?

Bound, trapped in a body in *shit* working order, reliant on me to lift cup to lips, fork to mouth, punch buttons on the TV remote, bossed and manhandled, how does David stand it? Well, he has to poor bugger, doesn't he?

No choice. That's on bad days and not every day is bad... Not *bad/ good* I correct myself, a *down* day, an *up* day.

His changing states, at a flip of some invisible switch, floor me. Add that how-to lesson to the syllabus, please.

... and when he was up he was up, and when he was down he was down, and when he was neither up nor down, I hum. How will I find him today?

Crises willing, me-with-me-alone-time is a few minutes each morning before breakfast.

The second I inhale my incense stick, light a puja candle, tap three rings to reverberate my singing bowl, tranquility settles. My meditation cushion placed just so, I watch dawn strike Santa Fe Baldy's distant mountain peak.

Birds like the chants I play, it seems, for I see them still on the bush outside the window, heads cocked. Twittering. Perhaps, like me, they gather their intention for the day and summon strength enough to follow through.

From a deep space, I feel the spirits of who it is I really am, who David really is, and see our earthly struggles as no more permanent than Hamlet's at London's Globe. I ponder the power of words, the tone in which they are uttered. I swear to let my speech pass through three gates before I ever speak. Remind myself,... *gentleness, patience, kindness.*

David is a perfect soul I have the honor to serve, I affirm.... *to treat as I would the Dali Lama, the Queen of England, Mohamed Ali or Pope Francis.*

Behind closed eyes, I draw in the beauty of the man I married. The great love we share. I am his. He is mine.

Calm settles for a few hours, a few days, a week or month. Whistled code-talk, singsong-messages, and love-hugs remind of happiness we share as man and wife.

Oh, dear, my finger hesitated over the keypad. SHARED? SHARE? Is happiness now relegated to the past?

I am grieving. I am in mourning.

5. think your home is your castle? think again

… not after you let them in… the skilled therapists and do-gooding friends. Those people *know* what's best for him.

Get it? I AM JUST HIS WIFE.

Demands couched politely, "I want you to… you must… you should… you've *got* to… ," sets my skin wrinkling.

Try asking, oh please, ask me, don't tell if you want me to do, to change home and habit.

My mouth zipped shut, I watch the social worker mark her list, assess me, our home and furniture, the needs of my husband, alarmed to realize she could declare our environment unsafe, and me unsuitable as his caregiver.

Whoa.

Is our home not our castle, and our choice to stay right here together and not have David carted off to some end of life facility our right?

So do I, or don't I want help? Problem. Of course I do. I'm a wreck when first my husband arrives home from hospital and pill-counting, safety and personal care scramble the hours.

Yet now, after we've begun to manage, I feel a victim of home invasion as a squadron of therapists swoop cheerfully past me through the front door headed for David's room.

Nurse, Physio, Occupational, Speech each therapist hammers their particular rules of therapy, and which home aids are musts.

MUST? Hmm. That word again.

"Now let me show you how to use… " I stare bemused at the sock-putter-on's tangle of plastic and tapes, the yoga belt, the lollipop sponge on a stick and the catalogue of unimaginables.

Pad handles on our cutlery? No thanks. Remove all floor rugs? No way. Surely is it is for David to adapt, learn to negotiate obstacles so he can safely visit other people's houses.

OK aids, the ones that make total sense: a wheelchair friendly flag-stone pathway from the garage to the front door; solar lamps to light the way; raised toilets; flexible shower head; grab-bars, suction mats and a bench in the shower; slip-trip proofed floor rugs; a swing table beside his favorite chair… now those I can take.

"This is a home not a clinic." I return their glares of disapproval.

Don't start me on the pros and cons of handicapped walking sticks… Same goes for the walker and the wheelchair. I'm not being awkward to be awkward. I want a say!

"They'll destroy his own sense of balance. While he can do without, he should." I retort. "Don't you think it a little premature? Counter productive, even?"

Use it or lose it, I maintain.

I refer to balance, walking, feeding, dressing, bathing, swimming, the whole gamut of skills needed to preserve independence. Give up swimming as the Senior Service Official said we should?

Absolutely not.

"So what if he freezes? He'll hardly drown where lifeguards are on duty, now will he?" I retort.

The Senior Services guy shook his head unconvinced. "Water is dangerous… "

He only need come to the class, see David roll and undulate free as a fish, see him spark alive in the warm water, kick and paddle arms and hands...

Three MUST USE aids, according to the helpers: walker, straps and sticks.

I stand by, watch the physio show how I MUST strap David with a yoga belt and grab him round his middle; how he MUST walk with a stick. It's not that I want David to trip, but is that any way to treat my husband? Any adult for that matter?

"Thanks but no thanks," I defend. "He walks perfectly well on his own. He's not a toddler," I reiterate.

Therapists are scared of being sued, I guess.

They give me a look, strap the belt around his middle anyway, gripping it from the back before marching him around the house.

Up and down the drive I try my best to demonstrate four-legged crab and horse gaits before encouraging him to try. But which leg to move with which stick was beyond the both of us. Legs and sticks intertwined tripping him — and me.

Stumbling sticks, we named them giggling, and dumped them in the umbrella stand.

The belt's off the second they drive away. We are too. David scuttling beside me a little lopsided, he walks to the end of our dirt drive unaided. Sunny afternoons, arm in arm, I guide his steps into the uneven arroyo of our village *bosque* and rest a moment beneath the Cottonwood's transfixed by the rustle of their leaves.

"The sea. Hear it?" David whispers. Breathing deeply we are still.

David is brave. David is strong. David lives everyday to the full. Me? I'm not so sure.

Caregivers and your Cared-for:
LEAP THE BARRIERS WHILE YOU CAN.

"This past summer holidaying in France where our family live,

David rode an Alpine chairlift."Disbelief clouds their eyes when I tell people. My son called up asking if handicapped people were allowed.

"Mais oui, but yes." We stop the lift, help him on and stop it again at the top.

Proof—the photo souvenir of David beside me our feet dangling over the treetops; the memory of the mountain picnic above a hidden lake; of returning after a short hike and finding him lopsided in a folding chair surrounded by cows curiously gazing; of the taste of wine and wildflower scented air, our lovely family.

David is brave. David is strong. David lives everyday to the full.

Me? I'm not so sure.

I have discovered your blog today. It helped me feel less lonely and what you write is so pertinent to my life. I relate to the 24 hours a day 'on duty'. I leave him only for half an hour at a time but have to get out or I will go mad. Everyone tells me I must take some respite, but I can't bring myself to do so yet. My body hurts from doing everything and my heart hurts with the sadness of it all. ~Carol

6. vision quest beyond the box
not yet a caregiver, i become his eyes

"My Owl," David, my husband, I catch him staring at me. His triple lenses diffuse pale discs of light.

"Well, what d'you see?" I quizzed.

"You. You can't imagine… now I know these glasses can't be right unless I'm in a house of mirrors," he giggled.

Moving towards me David crash-banged a side table so large I hadn't thought to cry a warning. An empty coffee mug skidded to the floor.

Lunching with friends just a week back, he carefully picked up the milk jug and poured its contents into the sugar bowl.

"Stop. Stop," I yell several times a day. "Too late. Too late."

In the golden years four years ago when the DBS was doing its thing and life was relatively normal, not yet a caregiver, not yet on overload, I took on the role as David's eyes.

"Step-alert. Down one. Two. Three to go. Watch out — pavement." I cried snatching his sleeve too late at as David air-stepped into the street.

"Danger. Danger."

The phone rang late one evening after a meal out.

"Did your husband intend to leave a $1,000 tip?" The manager checked. The receipt in David's pocket showed a scrawl of two extra unintended zeros.

More and more frequently I came home to find David sitting before a blank television screen, too ashamed to ask for help, the TV remote useless in his hand. Same problem with the phone.

"Can you dial for me? Can't make out a darn thing. All I get are wrong numbers and bleeps," he confessed.

"I am a blind man. I might as well cancel my New Yorker subscription. No point renting subtitled foreign films." David shook his head, defeated. He took to listening to tapes for the blind.

So-called specialists floundered flummoxed suggesting stronger prisms be added to his already thick lenses.

"Accept it," some sagely agreed. "Vision problems are to be expected of people suffering from Parkinson's Disease."

"Be grateful," the neurologist snapped sharply, "For seven years you've have been relatively tremor free thanks to the DBS implants."

What kind of answer was that? Nothing to do, but accept failing sight to the list of Parkinson's symptoms? Hmmm.

Then, *one fine day*, as many fairy tales begin…

It was during a rehab session after routine surgery for a new battery…

The Physio' working with him, and I, watched David, his careful placement of bricks midair entirely missing the target.

"I don't believe he can see," the Physio' said turning to me. "Have you ever considered working with an alternative ophthalmologist? There's one near you. I hear his results are amazing."

Swallowing my caustic, "No. Really? You mean he can't see? We've been trying to tell you specialists that for years," I almost kissed her feet.

"His approach is unusual," she hesitated. "Be warned."

Back home, googling his name, we watched an interview on YouTube,

"Nothing to lose but $$$," we decided. "Let's at least give it a go."

"Come in," the barefoot vision doctor's gentle voice invited.

Soft music played. The calm interior of the geodesic dome welcomed. Suspicious, I watched every move, noted the casual tracksuit he wore, the curious office space, the disproving shake of his head behind David's back as he observed David, silent, staring blankly at an electric-lit eye chart.

"Do you mind?" The doc inquired with a shiver, and replaced my husband's owl glasses with a pair of single-lens over the counter readers. "And now?"

"c.f.e.v.m... " David read from a page of large print. "Dog. Table. Ship... " Just like that.

Finally. Could this be, I smiled—someone who might help David SEE clearly again?

"Single magnification lenses are much easier for your eyes to deal with. Think of your poor, already compromised Parkinson's brain. How can it possibly know to which lens of your trifocals it should focus?"

"Now that made total sense," we nodded.

He kept talking, sharing his knowledge.

"I believe in brain and eye muscles re-education, not complicated prescription glasses. ... re-awaken the body's own bio-intelligence... "

So simple a concept. On the spot we agreed to six bi-weekly sessions and committed to practicing between visits as he insisted I work alongside David.

"You too," he turned to me. "A little every day. The idea is to attempt the task, not to do it perfectly."

Seemingly a little whacky and nothing to do with eyes, we hummed, made faces, moved our limbs, lips and tongue.

"To stimulate energy meridians and ventricles in the brain, because... " he explained, "the retina, is part of the brain."

"Catch." I threw a ball to David.

"Catch." He threw it back.

Our normally tidy living room turned into a playground of bouncing balls, card games and floating juggling scarves. Charts and newspaper headlines littered the table.

"A. Z. C." We sang out letters from newspaper headlines to the beat of a metronome while wobbling heel-toe between the floor tiles.

Our grey matter stretched with crazy-making mind-gymnastics.

Kindergarten all over again, we played. I'd forgotten how. Became rivals, as in our younger tennis and squash days, the 'US' we used to be. David's old self, my companion, husband, glimmered.

"Ready for a game of... ?" David initiated many exercises himself.

Me-caregiver, you-patient shook loose. I could step back. Laugh. Be silly. Have fun. I could see the difference in David's body:mind:eye co-ordination, and memory skills. I heard it in his voice. Then one day...

"What the devil... ?"

I caught sight of David's half-clothed form streaking through the house.

"You didn't know I could run did you?" He laughed vanishing into his den.

Six months passed, it happened.

"Hey, I can read."

He reeled off sentences from the book on his lap, his face shining. As though to prove it to himself, he read out paragraph after paragraph. "I might paint, I might even drive again," he added.

But we're human. We got lazy. The newness wore off. Daily exercising slipped to occasional not because of disinterest, but for our lack of energy and motivation. Like renovating a house. You do enough to make it habitable, but never get round to the finishing touches.

I couldn't get him going and I wasn't about to force him. Plain tired of that role.

"Ah. I was waiting for you to bring that up... " the vision doctor pounced on the fifth session. "At our first meeting I saw David's life-force was severely depleted but until you recognized it there was no point addressing the problem — oxygenate and re-vitalize his body."

The breathing exercises, dietary changes, supplements combined with the other tasks did something. David now climbed out of the exercise pool rejecting the chair lift; swinging his arms he strode to the mailbox. I watched him, an apple in hand headed for the neighbor's horse.

Up. Down. Up Down. David demonstrated standing, sitting from a low chair at the Neurologists office,

"Wow. Just look at you move," she exclaimed scribbling on her chart. "You don't present as a Parkinson's Patient today. It's working whatever it is you are doing."

It's not to say David is without disability. He is. Some days are depressingly bad. For him. For me. Our frustration with the slow grind of progress in mastering the simplest task.

No wonder he's lost enthusiasm. No wonder he's fed up adjusting focus along a knotted length of string. Take his E-reader — one tremor and the page disappeared, sent him right back to the beginning.

Tired, his voice fades infuriatingly inaudible. Or worse, he never makes a sound and I can't tell if he just can't or just won't answer me.

Example: "Would you like eggs or cereal and fruit today for break-fast?" No response, the question hangs unanswered. "I'm waiting, I'm waiting. Will you ANSWER," I finally lose it.

Example: Mouth breathing, he lolls tilted sideways in his chair, gazes at the flickering television screen for hour upon hour till I could scream. And do sometimes. My favorite cry: "Your brain will ROT."

Not nice of me I know, but supposedly I am human. I can't tell him I'm dying inside, ripped apart imagining the terror I know he feels but doesn't voice, the terror of being sucked down by Parkinson's—S-L-O-W-L-Y. My creeping fears are wisps of vapor by comparison. I force them under wraps.

Looking on the bright side good things have stayed—like not knocking into obstacles because he *sees* them, and giving back the taped books for the blind because he can read depending on the size and density of the print.

Sitting side by side on the balcony in Puerto Vallarta's sunshine, our noses deep in printed worlds, our sighs melded with the gentle waves. He devoured three paperbacks in as many weeks.

Three year's ago we took a drive to Bosque Del Apache wetlands.

The sun shone. Entering the sanctuary, the lake's surface appeared to lift as hundreds of migrating snow geese took to the air. Back and over, around and around, they dipped and brushed the water again and again. Leaning backwards across the car's hood, David marveled at the yellow feet tucked beneath the white of their wings, a white made more brilliant by the backdrop of a cloudless sky.

Stopping at an observation deck the mounted binoculars trained on the skeleton of a lone tree across the water. Perched on a branch I picked out a large bird with my naked eye—white cowl and trouser legs, yellow talons and beak, it turned its head to face me.

"Quick, quick, David there, there," I pointed.

David located the tree, pressed his glasses close to the binoculars' eyepiece, and gasped.

"An eagle. I can see an eagle."

December16, 2017

7. cats in the belfry

READY FOR THE CATS, CAREGIVERS?

Better check the small print on medications. Use a spy-glass to reveal what drug companies hope we'll never see.

… in some cases … hallucinations may occur. Right.

No good expecting your doctor to point out side effects, it's another task relegated to us caregivers. "PROACTIVE," is the buzzword.

"There. See it? The cat. It's run under the table. Oh look another jumped on the chair. And there and there."

A psychiatrist in his working life, if anyone could recognize a hallucination it was David. Those cats at least.

"Look," David remarked during breakfast. "What on earth are those children in swimsuits doing round the bird feeder in our garden?"

"They are but wisps of your imagination gone wild." I smiled. His expression showed he didn't quite believe me. "Where, exactly?" I asked. Tell me what they're doing now."

"They run and hide if I look for them."

His neurologist astonished me by giggling and looking around the cluttered space when I told her.

"Do you see any cats now, here in my office?"

"Just a white one." David cocked his head in its direction of her file cabinet.

"If they don't bother you David, then leave the cats be." She smirked.

He saw horses one time. Herds. Crowding the fence by the road, galloping up the drive.

His illusionary images were no bother. Linked to a particular antibiotic the last dose sent the cats packing. We'd grown used to them. Knew they were harmless.

Not so fifteen years back when hallucinations first invaded his perception. That golden decade after his DBS — deep brain implants — zero-ed his tremor, tucked Parkinson's into the back alleyways of our minds.

I was a wife then, and he, David, my husband. Normal. Oblivious of Parkinson's shadowing our lives, we lived to travel, experience cultures unlike our own — the Americas, Europe, India and Sri Lanka. Medication — the only reminder of the PD burden we packed with us on those vacations.

During a week's stop-over in London en-route to Sri Lanka, we stayed in our son's house, and woke one morning to spaghetti strings stuck to the wall and tomato paste-smeared pans littering the kitchen — evidence of wild midnight feasting.

The following night the same scene, and the next.

"I believe David is sleepwalking," our daughter-in-law surmised. "Maybe it's the stress of travel."

E-m-b-a-r-e-s-s-i-n-g, but not alarming.

Then I caught him standing in the bedroom with a coat hanger swinging on his arm.

"What the hell… ?" I gasped.

"Don't you know," earnest, he turned to me., "it's the new way to take blood pressure?"

"Don't be daft. Why not stand on your head as well?" I laughed to cover a creeping fear. Was senility setting in?

I didn't recognize it then, the first taste of what lay ahead. David and I, our roles switched. Me — Tarzan. David — Jane.

Blinkered to all but following our travel plan, I waved away the incidents as no more important than a hiccup. Nothing a good night's sleep wouldn't right, we all of us agreed.

I can't believe it never occurred to me to take his nocturnal forays seriously. After all, I reasoned, once we arrived in Sri Lanka, what with the sun, sightseeing, relaxing, David would soon be himself.

And he was at first. We walked the Galle seafront, people watched, and crashed a Hindu wedding celebration at our hotel.

It's too long ago to remember every incident. Blanked them out if I'm honest. He began doing crazy stuff like spraying shaving foam onto the mirror, and speaking oddly to imaginary people. But what to do so far from home?

One taxi drive sticks in my mind. Tilting precariously from an open-sided Tuk-tuk into the traffic lane of whizzing trucks and buses, I begged him, tugging at his arm.

"Please, David, lean back in. You'll get hit." It was as if I hadn't spoken. He just wouldn't right himself upright. Taking charge, I yelled yanking on his arm and pulled him out of danger.

Then dining one evening in a frangipani scented garden, I no longer recall exactly what he said, only that his rambling frightened me. Something about me being a circus performer and wanting to get married.

"Huh? You're burbling. Want a second wedding? Are you a little drunk?" I parried.

Two days later, barefoot, I trod in a puddle where he'd peed yellow rivers against our bedroom wall, woken me with its streaming.

"Deep down you must hate me," I whimpered.

"Of course not, silly goose," he kissed my eyelids. "I must have been sleep-walking."

The following two weeks David was David again. Happy tourists, we walked to a muddy river with the herd in Pindewalla's elephant orphanage, listened to the clacking of giant bamboo in Mountbatten's botanical gardens, glimpsed Bhudda's tooth in Kandy, drove through ancient fern trees, clambered Sigiriya's two thousand year-old archaeological site guided by our Sri Lankan friend, glorying in his country.

Over lunch one day, the two of us alone in Galle, David leaned across the table, urged,

"Look. Behind you — those people in formal evening dress with ice skates on their heads."

"They've gone now," I comforted.

"That's it… David's going insane. Now what? Don't panic. Don't panic," I panicked. Choices scrambled.

Should I evacuate him back to the US in a straight jacket, sign him into a local psychiatric hospital… ? My first taste of taking charge, and I had no solution.

"Calm. Be calm," I told myself, "Meditate." Cross-legged quietly on my bed I shut my eyes, prayed to all the Gods that ever lived. "Help me, my sweet lover is drowning in a cerebral sea."

An unseen angel whispered, "Check his medication."

I bowed my head, waited for a lucid moment to tell my madman he was mad. I took his hands,

"Pretend," I told my husband, "You are the doctor. Your patient is behaving oddly."

He fell silent, checked the phial's smallest print … *in some cases… hallucinations may occur.*

Pill by pill, day by day, cutting his medication, my David returned to earth.

✳   ✳   ✳

Rolling, rolling, rolling... Yippee ayaaa... The decade I call our Parkinson's golden years cruised by — the time between having his implants, and when e-coli infection sent him spiraling.

Nothing remarkable stands out but a little aging. I was happy in my studio tramping clay beneath my feet, and pounding out and firing my sculptures uninterrupted by *can you help me please* calls from David.

His implanted batteries died every two or three years necessitating surgery under a general anesthetic to replace them and the connecting wires.

"What?" I asked incredulously, "We can send a man into space yet can't recharge an implanted battery without carving into a person's body?"

Routine. A nuisance. Non life-threatening hospital stays were a part of life. The last was different. Seven or eight months passed.

David felt a damp spot behind his ear at the site where two wires connected beneath the skin. Alarm bells rang. e-coli infection. Rushed for immediate surgery to remove the wire and battery pack and prevent the killer infection traveling to his brain. The heavy antibiotic prescribed — intravenously at first, followed by a further six weeks — would stamp out the last of the e-coli.

Back home, all was well until one night.

"Get UP. Get up. Quick," David shook me from sleep tugging at my sheets, his voice urgent, his eyes, tiger-wild. "We must leave now before the firemen get here. They're coming to torch our house."

He gripped my arm pulling me towards the front door. His strength, superhuman, I had no choice.

The car keys dangled on the hook. *If he sees them we are done... If he reaches the door...*

"Wait. Wait," I stalled. "Let me get my dressing gown. The police have told us we must sit tight, and wait for instructions. We have to wait here for their call, or they won't be able to find us." I lied.

"You're right," he hesitated... "but, be ready to go."

"Let's have a cup of tea until they arrive. Here..." My voice trembled.

Pretending calm, terror spun words from my mouth. Soothing. Adrenaline saved me where reason and resistance would have failed.

I held the phone, my finger poised to punch in 911. One step towards the door and I would dial. We sipped in silence. Drained our mugs.

"I feel like going back to bed... are you ready yet?" My voice low, I took his hand.

"O.K." he said.

And that was that. Well not quite. Maybe for him. I lay shivering till dawn re-ran the psychotic scenario time and again, straining for any sound but for snoring from his room. Plotted how to catch him before he slipped away.

Take warning caregivers. Side effects can harm even kill.

Mostly Doctors don't want to scare us, put ideas into our heads.

"It's rare but let me know of any reaction to the medication," might be the closest to listing what could go wrong..

... *could cause liver failure... heart attack... suicidal thoughts... muscle wasting.,* murmur the TV advertisements.

"And you want me to ingest what?" I yell at the screen.

"Yeah, baby. What... like a psychotic hallucination?"

Now that is what I call a reaction. Wouldn't you?"

I repeat, CHECK THE SMALL PRINT.

8. "en guard, messieurs"
dare me... cross this line

"My civil rights are being invaded." His words.

His custodian, duty demands I, his wife and caregiver, keep him off society's scrap heap. Fight on his behalf. Protect. Defend.

I learned how at age six in the land of my birth, India. My loving Ayah disappeared. My mother and half-sister too. No explanation. There one day, gone the next. The British Courts dragged me and my baby brother away and into the care of strangers. Months later my father appeared. With my arms wrapped around my brother, we were shipped to England, and dumped abandoned in a children's home until I was almost eleven. Walnut hard mantling a vulnerable interior nobody, but nobody saw inside my shell. I made sure of that. I am that tough-nut person once again. Have to be.

"En guard, messieurs," I prepare for battle, brandish my foil.

I pinched my arm. Proved I was ready to fend the missiles aimed at David, me, our space. When I played Lacrosse at boarding school in Goalie position, just the same. Thwack. In terror of injury, I lobbed back the hail of balls before they ever struck my face and padded body-armor. Now, as David's advocate, the same. Thwack. Thwack.

For two agonized days after a fall, David allowed no EMT near.

Be prepared caregivers, its our loved ones right to refuse resuscitation and may seize the opportunity to exit earth.

"What if your hip is broken, I find you unconscious, have pneumonia, a heart attack... what shall I tell the EMTs? Make you comfortable and leave, or take you to hospital?" I pressed. No answer. Pain, the clincher, forced his choice.

"Call 911. I need to go to the ER," David pleaded. Saved his life as it turned out.

Apart from a fractured vertebrae, tests revealed bi-lateral pulmonary embolisms caused from hours of sitting on our recent Trans Atlantic flight—another task for caregivers: nag your loved one to pump those legs and stamp those feet every hour you're in the air.

I could work just as well on my laptop in his hospital room as well as anywhere, I convinced myself. And for the next week hunkered down beside his bed for six, seven hours. Just as well. One morning arriving at ten, I found him defeated, slumped forgotten, unwashed, un-fed in a grubby, un-made bed. New temporary nurses shrugged when I complained.

"He's supposed to be dressed and sitting in a chair. Doctor's orders," I admonished.

"It's good to have an advocate," the on-call neurologist approved when I complained. Yeah. But what if I hadn't been there? The light was already out in David's eyes.

There's a battle yet to come.

David's discharge looming, three-weeks in-patient rehab was arranged—not to the hospital's in-house unit as I requested, but to a facility for the desperate.

"David failed to meet the necessary requirements,"

The physio therapist squirmed. Tall and blonde, he forced a smile. "He'll be transferred to a residential home. Yesterday your husband only walked ten paces, and to qualify he must show improvement every day. That's the protocol."

"Protocol be damned... And do you know why he only took ten steps?" I sneered. "Maintenance taped his door to keep him in his room because the hallway was being waxed. I insist he be re-assessed." One look at me, and they agreed.

With four hours of therapy daily, I watched him claim back his functions over the next week until...

... one afternoon visit ten days into his stay, David's eyes swiveled upwards, to the window sill, and from wall to wall, "Look — white cats. See them? There's another and another. What am I doing here in a cattery?"

I froze, frantic. One back-slip and he'd be expelled from the program.

I dashed home, and with a psych-nurse friend checked his patient portal. Yesterday's urine tests: abnormal, abnormal—every one. An infection — oh Praise the Lord. He wasn't bonkers. I exploded in tears.

"You're mistaken. His tests were normal," Dr. White-Coat in charge contradicted. "No sign of infection."

Wrong. Wrong. Did I have to fight every inch to prove it? "See — it's written—yesterday." I jabbed my finger at the date.

White-coat disappeared. Returned with his head hung low having double-checked the lab's report. I'll give him that.

"I owe you a big apology."

Granted a reprieve, David stayed. But what about computer-illiterates, those without computers wrongly diagnosed with no-one to speak for them, those unfortunates carted off to end-of-life homes where they should never be?

So toughen up, sharpen your swords caregivers, it's up to us to fight.

The 20 days in rehab allowed by Medicare was up.

"We want him admitted into a residential home for four weeks. He is not ready to go home." Not a question, a pronouncement.

"Further therapy... " they said.

"Further therapy?" I snorted, for I knew therapy in the facility they suggested happened maybe ten minutes a couple of times a week if that. And worse as a "fall risk," tied down to his bed attached to an alarm forbidden to visit even the toilet un-escorted, he'd lose his strength to walk.

"He'll turn up his toes and die in there. I'm taking him home. Medicare covers twenty home visits — a nurse, physio, O.T., and speech therapy. He'll get all the help he needs."

Buttoning my ears, I hinted at the patient's right to self discharge. Reluctantly Big-Chief-White-Coat agreed I could take him home. "On condition you have round the clock help for him, and the caregiver completes an hour's safety training with the unit's Physiotherapist."

Problem. Excepting me — no caregiver. I wracked my brains, re-membered a friend. He'd looked after an elderly man for years till relatives hauled the poor chap off to end his days in residential care. No way would I let that happen to David.

"Can you help me?" I begged my friend. "Pretend you are David's caregiver."

A perfect actor, he donned a white coat and trained with the phys-io. Freed from the ward's clutches stifling our giggles, we whisked David up, up, up and away. I slipped a couple of tens into my friend's pocket at the curbside, hugged, and fled.

Home-alone, now what to do? I stared at the box of shots given me by the hospital. "Twice a day for ten days... nothing to it," they waved me away.

Miraculous fluke: my GP brother-in-law and sister from Oaklahoma happened by unexpectedly en-route to California. Demonstrating how to pinch David's belly flesh and stab, I winced and plunged the needle.

Having him back home was a gift. David had no need to say it, gladness, relief, happiness sparkled in his eyes. I crawled into bed beside him burrowing beneath the duvet. How lucky we were.

"Night, night darling. Sleep well." We both did.

December 31, 2016

9. Like it or no Prepare to Play God

I blame his French friend for his decline, her overprotectiveness in not allowing him to get up from his chair, or let him walk a step without rushing to clutch his arm.

"I 'elp you." Her accented voice grates.

'Elp, my arse, I cursed. Pinpoint his spiral from alert communicator to silent partner to his fall, the tumble she caused that day.

Mid summer with our family in the French Alps, David and I, on a day's outing to medieval La Roche sur Foron, met up with an old friend of David's. Well, long-time-back ex-girlfriend, to be honest. No wonder she annoyed the hell out of me.

"It's better he relies on his own balance," I suggested politely seeing her grip his arm. I glared, too damn British to tell her, "Leave him be." For that I kick myself.

SPEAK YOUR MIND.

TRUST YOUR INSTINCT KNOWS. I wish I had.

The look she gave me... my mouth clamped shut... should have insisted, pulled him from her, grabbed his other arm. Something. God, if I could go back... She meant well of course. I've forgiven her — almost — but cannot quite rinse away the bitter taste of blame, the what-if scenario...

We'd barely taken a step, me leading, the two of them behind me chattering together not looking where they were going, when crash, head first, the granite post demarking the town square spun him bloodied to the ground. Sliced his leg clear to the bone.

No good being squeamish, I took a breath, held the two flaps of flesh together across his shin till the *Pompier* arrived bells clanging.

David's friend rode and sat five hours with me in the ER. Never once apologized. Never a hint of admitting fault.

HERS

Though the injury was no deeper than the dozen stitches embroidering his leg, shocked, his body's systems collapsed.

First his bladder quit, a week later his bowels.

"Trauma can do that to someone with Parkinson's," the doctor explained.

David's third visit to the ER, signaled — no, not the end — the beginning of the downward spiral of his mind and body, and my true start to full time caregiving.

I donned a CAREGIVER'S HAT for real. Upended my life. Faced another.

Job description… change and cleanse body parts and catheter bags, help him sit and stand, push arms into sleeves, feet into shoes, prevent his stumble, count pills… overcome my resistance. And yes, occasional revulsion. Oh indeed, the caregiver's hat pinched.

"Will the TSA allow him to travel wearing a catheter?" I worried. "What about the ban on liquids?"

I insisted the doctor give me an OK-to-travel chit.

With no lurching from seat to the airplane *lavs,* no chance of getting stuck inside, the catheter made for easier travel.

David bore — wore — the thing for nearly two years. Caused so many infections and episodes of brain-fog, we lost count.

"I'm losing it. I can't remember numbers any more... and... " David's sentence hung unfinished.

His body tired, too many hours passed asleep where he sat. His will sapped, television's white noise took the place of friends. His six-foot spine began its curve and dropped the top of his head level with my chin never again to tower above me, for my lips to reach for his.

If all that wasn't enough for us both to deal with, his eyes often froze shut rendering him blind and needing me to steer him around the furniture and corners of our house.

The balance tipped. More and more frequently David slipped out of reach into Parkinson's cruel sea. Wife made way for caregiver.

The following year the worst happened.

In the French mountain village staying with our family again, Septic Shock felled David into violent seizures and unconsciousness.

It's hard to go back to that night, his body jerking, his struggle for life. Surreal images flash.

Eight EMTs' rubber boots tramping across our double bed to reach him, their walkie-talkies crackling instructions, Miles, Kate, and me helpless in the doorway, the scrambled bag-packing and dressing, my overpowering thirst for tea, tea and more tea, the endless two hour pacing while the doctor worked to stabilize him enough to survive the ambulance ride.

In the US no doctor would have visited in the dead of night. But for the eight EMTs and trauma doctor David would be gone.

Miles and I hunched wordless in a locked hospital waiting room. No thoughts. Three. Four Five a.m... The door opened and we were ushered into another windowless room.

Kleenex box. Bad sign. I noticed it immediately on the table before we sat. I felt nothing, said not a word, watched my hands clasp my son's, the two faces across from me float disembodied, not sure if I was awake.

A thought blinded, "He's gone." A second flashed, "I'm a widow."

"Your husband is alive right now but he will die in a couple of hours if we don't treat him immediately. Do we have your permission to go ahead?" The English-speaking doctor's voice knifed the silence.

"But what of his Medical Directive? His wishes? We made an agreement... never... a vegetable," my words stumbled.

They scrutinized the document I handed them.

"Treatment for e-coli infection is a medical, so does not go against the DO NOT RESUCITATE conditions. Once the infection is under control, he should fully recover and be able to breathe on his own in about a week. If not, you and I can have another conversation."

A hurried whisper between my son and I... should I, shouldn't I... ?

To die so traumatized, so unprepared, so not at peace was no way to go. How would his spirit ever rest? Did he want me to let him die? Would he forgive me if he was forced to keep living?

I couldn't deny him this one last chance, I just couldn't.

I chose LIFE.

But had I? Five days he lay in a coma.

"Had I done wrong?" I wept, my head buried in my family's arms.

BE PREPARED TO PLAY GOD, caregivers.

I carry our DNR documents with me when we travel. To the grocery store even. Another hangs on the refrigerator. Being told is not enough, EMTs and emergency room doctors must see the legal document or they are obligated to do all they can to save their client. Neither of us wants to be resuscitated, so the DNR is not something we want to be caught without.

The doctors forecast right.

Day six. There David sat in bed detached from tubes, pink cheeked, propped up — an angel in his pale blue gown.

Son, daughter in law, granddaughter and me, suited up in our throw-aways — gowns, masks, gloves and over shoes — ran crying to his side. He, we, beaming, so happy.

Few nurses spoke English. His new ward Isolation became a prison. Locked. The hospital doors swung open on the dot of 2pm. Closed at 6 sharp. Bedridden, days stretched. To sixteen.

death sits in his eyes in the rustle of the leaves
outside his hospital window-waits to claim his
frail body-waits for his soul to drop its hold.

I wrote this while he slept. Another week had passed. Recovery yawned with no end date ahead.

"I can't go through this again. I am too weak," tears spilled onto his cheeks. "I have no strength to even try. Promise you won't let them force me to stay alive. I just want to die," he whispered.

"I want this to be my last day. I'm filled with love for you, but I'm begging you, get me moved to palliative care where I can die in peace. Last night I vowed to forever refuse food and drink, but the nurses forced me to eat. I am so helpless."

Wife's? Advocate's? God's? Whose hat to wear?

I stroked his hand. Comforted him. Prayed for guidance. Death. Liberation. Fate. God's plan. David's right to choose. Subjects we'd already discussed the previous summer, so when THE difficult subject re-surfaced, the choice to die, the right to die with dignity, I had some idea of David's wishes.

The French hospital lay ten miles from Geneva's DIGNITAS, Switzerland's suicide clinic and a legal medically assisted end. I "googled" for information.

By the time I researched the organization's hows and whats, David recovered enough to revise plans. He decided to die back in the

USA under hospice care if he could survive that long.

"Give a good-bye party, then slip away." He recited the names of friends and family to be invited, and who was to have this picture, that ring.

"Have you ordered the pine box?" He asked another day.

"The only way home is business class or in an urn on my lap," I flipped the serious question unsure. Was he joking.? Would he see home alive?

He did. He made it. A medical assistant and me by his side, he landed safely at Albuquerque's Sunport, New Mexico. Thank God for travel insurance. They paid.

My God-role was not yet over. Though the sun shone a little brighter every day, I lost hope when he announced,

"I need you to contact the Hemlock Society… in case I choose to take the next step. I'll be gone by the New Year."

Wrong. The leaflets I downloaded from my computer lie in a file unopened beside my heart.

Nothing prepares us caregivers for the agony of choice.

David put off his goodbye party till Christmas three months away. Winter solstice arrived, and with its passing death retreated. The New Year, then his January birthday surprised him.

In the falling quiet of snow, the pecking of a red-breasted finch seeking seed, and the dogged persistence of migrating Canadian geese headed for southern feeding grounds, our world began to spin again as David strove to live.

As for me, unlike Humpty Dumpty, I gathered up the pieces and glued myself together.

10. 'tis the season to be JOLLY...

Not as a caregiver it isn't. People want UP and happy-clappy not DOWN. Party season only accentuates society's banishment, our isolation.

And I have to admit the word *jolly* does not describe David.

"Good party. I had a great time," he smiles un-fazed from sitting alone, slumped eye level with guests' belly buttons circling around him.

Not me. I butterfly from and towards him poised to dive for his plate, his glass before its contents hit the floor, tense, unable to em-merse myself in the bright fun.

David and partying are just not on.

Unlike a couple of years ago when we looked forward to a crowded calendar during party season and village neighbors included us in the social whirl, I am now a stay-at-home. Like it too.

Could be a crafty defense tactic against pain of rejection — yes, I give you that — but truly I choose our own fireside twosome any day to battling the scrum while forking pasta salads and such, bellowing.

"Sorry. Can't hear a word. Again, what did you say?" A lively dis-cussion around the table with intelligent friends, a glass of wine in hand and plates of scrumptious food — well, OK, OK, those dinner parties I do miss. Some at least.

It's happening — David's and my withdrawal from society.

I sense its creeping as I fall into my slops each evening with my hair un-brushed, permit bottled mayo and plastic containers on the dining table, finger-licking and shameful to admit, pour our breakfast coffee into yesterday's unwashed cup. Too plain uncivilized for the public, I get it. With nobody to see or *tut-tut*, who cares?

Strange, this story I wrote a year ago. "HER WAY OF TELLING IT," illustrates the crossroads where David and I stand today. I could have titled it "MY WAY... " but the word my grates uncomfortably too personal. It's a fable really, about two bees. My way of dealing with what I couldn't yet face.

HER WAY OF TELLING IT

It's been twenty years since the doctor in him died, since he shut himself inside the hive and made it his home. Sited on a rise among the purple flowering cholla, from the hive's opening he could see the sunrise spark Baldy Mountain's snow peak fifty miles away, and watch the moon slide her light into the sky those nights he was wakeful.

Standing in a shaft of dust motes he counted his sprouting bee parts. He didn't have to beg his wife to join him she just followed him inside and exchanged her dress for a fuzzy yellow pantsuit with black stripes.

"For better or worse," she pronounced, "I'm here for you." She popped a glob of pollen under her tongue puckering her lips.

With nobody to upbraid them, the couple let things slide. Beds stayed unmade, unwashed dishes stacked precariously beside the sink, and newspapers littered the floor or crammed the hollow spaces of the honeycomb long abandoned by the hive's previous occupants.

Of an evening, over a glass of dandelion or elderberry wine they laughed out loud pointing at the mess.

"Oh B-darling, she called him by his new nickname, how even one year ago we'd have died of shame."

To make the point, she spat out a sunflower husk and shuffled it with her foot onto the pile collecting on the floor.

The first two years of retirement they were able to hide out while they figured ways to adapt to a new way of living.

"We taking a long road trip," they lied to their friends.

The two of them mapped out a plan while their transformation took place — the time between human and bee when Dr. B's stomach-fur hadn't quite grown in, and wing buds still irritated Mrs. Bee's skin.

Though they pretended not to, their close friends noticed — physical and behavioral changes — the new roundness of their bodies, glazed pupils, difficulty forming words, sudden reluctance to shake hands or exchange hugs, and outright refusal to give out their new address. When they did leave the house, they enveloped their fur, their extra legs and budding wings with padded jackets, added at least ten pounds to their appearance.

"My, don't we look plump." They laughed poking a finger at the other's midriff.

It was one Saturday in February — the last time they

ventured out socially.

*"We won't take no for an answer. We insist you come,"
their good friends persuaded. "Rabbie Burns night. A
friend is bringing his bagpipes."*

*Their hosts ignored their sloppy manners, his tremor-
ing, the spilled innards of the haggis and gravy from
his fork, the petit pois rolling across the table, the slosh
of whiskey Dr B spattered on the cloth as the flaming
haggis was piped in.*

*Staring at the stubble sprouted on the doctor's chin,
their hostess marveled at how well they both looked, and
the elegance of their matching black and lemon-yellow
outfits.*

*"You look just like a pair of ... " Her smile smudged.
She ran her hand over her hair pushing away a strand
of unwanted sentence and stared at a cobweb cornered
by the ceiling.*

*Dr. B and Mrs. Bee caught one another' eyes. Though
brief, the exchange told the other they could no longer
risk exposure. Be seen in public.*

*The hum-mmm-ming surging from inside Dr. B
thrummed audible.*

*"Lovely evening. Thank you. We need to be going." It
was early but they wanted to be alone.*

*Next morning the shine of their black fur had dulled
to patchy tufts. The woman inspected her husband.
Slumped, his face almost touched the tablecloth. A fork
loaded with fried egg frozen in his right hand where
she'd forced it. Who knew how long he'd stay like that if
she let him. She heard a car drive up.*

*She roused him, helped him off with his bee suit.
Took off her own.*

11. heLLo! heLLo? anyone home?

Anybody home?

It's lonely here outside your world. I trace your profile with my gaze, the familiar silhouette on the pillow beside me for more than thirty years.

One room, two chairs we sit together of an evening in the rumble of television's tunnel journeying ever closer to a mysterious world beyond our own. I would prefer music, scrabble, conversation. Head back, jaw slack I notice his eyes are tight shut.

"Open your eyes darling," I encourage. "How can you possibly know what in God's name is going on? "

I don't understand why him watching television through closed eyelids should that bother me, but it does.

"Beam in Scotty," I joke, desperate to bring David back.

On good days the cracked vessel in which David resides releases the smart adolescent and child psychiatrist, the man he was, the man I married, my lover-husband and best friend, and we swap chit-chit before he sank turtle-like beneath the waves.

Has he even heard me, the stories I tell him, my questions?

"David, David, I'm talking to you." Words roam, no sign of landing in his mind.

Is David—anybody—there? And if there is, is he who he was, or the he who he is now? The question tumbles many times a day. Each time, my answer shifts. All I know is I am lonely and miss him.

"Be thankful you still have him. You will miss him more when he is gone," I tell myself, the breath of his human form, the endless chores of tending, the opportunity of purpose.

I see myself padding the vacuum of this empty house oppressed by unnatural silence. His chair vacant, I eat alone.

I watch the effort of his emerging the crumpled human slumped voiceless on his dining room chair each breakfast, the snail energy it takes to pop back from inside his shell.

By increments his head realigns with his neck. He snap-traps the drool sliding from the left corner of his slackened lips, retracts his left arm, always his left, through the armrest and creeps his blood-swollen fingers on the tablemat searching for his fork. His eyes are still shut, you see. He relies on feel.

No warning, without reason, all of a sudden, the David I married is back.

"Coffee please… ," Breakfast carries on as if he never *went*. "I'd like the marmalade, please. Do we have any plans for today?"

"He's like a sea turtle," I describe him to friends, "sinking then surfacing to life."

Anybody home, I wonder of my David, the times he switches off.

It could be minutes, half an hour or more, I find him, a statue frozen in mid-action sitting on his bed or chair, a sock dangling from his hand. Sometimes I catch him standing immobile, his face pushed against the wall. Can he hear or see me? There is no way I can get him to respond.

Take today, Tuesday.

Breakfast over, well the eating part of breakfast, David flopped over with his face on the plate. I have given up trying to bully him to sit up. It's best to leave him till he re-surfaces. When he's that switched off there is nothing I can do.

I cleared the table as best I could. Reaching awkwardly into a low cupboard, I lost my balance sending the butcher's cart flying and me crashing to the floor. I hurt mostly from shock of landing on my back. Did David stir, raise his head? Not a muscle.

What if I really hurt myself, fell unconscious, I worry. How long would the two of us be alone inside our walls? This morning's minor mishap is a wake-up call, one I've not yet thought through.

"Ah, he refuses to wear one of those press-button gizmos round his neck," I second-guess the unspoken solution you're offering me.

"If not him, then YOU wear one," a voice whispers.

It's a consideration I don't much like the thought of, but I get the point.

I shudder when I recall Christmas two years ago. Speed-walking to catch the propane truck, I tripped and did a *Stephen-Hawking-flat-faced-smack* into the paving stones. Wham.

Blood. Twisted limbs. Agony. Knocked momentarily to another world, my screams blended with the truck's roar and gas hiss, and I lay there unheard. When the delivery men finally heard my "Help. Help" and carried me inside, David never raised his head.

I push that example away... too painful to face. Could I bleed and DIE, the house go up in flames and still he wouldn't notice? The thought puts me in mind of our holiday in Mexico three year's ago.

David stretched out on the sofa, me on the balcony tapping away engrossed in what I was writing. Seeking the perfect word I raised my head. Black clouds of smoke billowed from the French doors obscuring the room beyond.

Inside three-foot flames licked the extraction hood above the stove eight feet from David.

"David. David. Get out the room's on fire." And rushing in I yelled,

"Get up. Get help. Quickly. Quickly."

Struggling from the couch he made for the door, while I slammed a saucepan lid over part of the blaze—my bag of teas, spices, punched the phone to summon help.

"Reception. How may I help you?" The hotel operator drawled. "Now? Would you like someone to come up?"

"Yes. Yes. Immediately." Was the woman nuts? Nobody appeared.

Then the greatest luck, two cleaners and a maintenance man happening by, rushed in and took control. Within half an hour the flames were doused, the smoke stains scrubbed and cinders thrown away along with the blackened toaster, extractor hood and frying pan.

Oh the shame. It was me. My fault. I had switched on the burner beneath a bagged stash of precious teas, spices and special treats brought from home.

tomorrow when I lie alone
when I have no shirts of his to wash
when I clear one plate from the table
when the back porch swings empty
I will wish…
I will weep
stare into the laundry basket
seek his pair of shorts to add
search in vain for his missing sock
I'll not complain
today I swear
promise only kindness
grumbling no more at
his snoring snuffling sleep
happy to still have him

January 21, 2017

12. the blue hole... 90 miles ahead

Driving home from a blogging class in Albuquerque one day last fall I passed a billboard on Route 66.

"LESS THAN TWO HOURS TO YOUR JOURNEY'S END. THE BLUE HOLE — 90 MILES AHEAD" proclaimed the advertisement of the local tourist attraction where without success scuba divers have sought its end.

The image of swimming through the Blue Hole's watery lens to infinity put me in mind of death.

Can you imagine, Caregivers, knowing your journey's end? Would knowing be a death sentence or relief? I imagined life shrinking, crossing off each day until none remained but one final sunset before embarking on a private mystery journey.

Would we, should we, weep for another year of life gone by? 10-9-8 — as we do when the New Year's ball begins its drop, then exchange kisses and rejoice...

HAPPY NEW YEAR. HAPPY NEW LIFE.

I imagine the agony of the terminally ill sentenced to a certain number of days of life, a prisoner counting hours one by one to–barbaric murder to my mind–execution.

I can't decide if knowing would collapse the two of us crazy with grief, or cinch us more tightly to each other. I can't decide if I would cram our last days doing all the things we'd wished to do but have never done.

My wish: hold hands with David watching dawn streak crimson-gold over the Taj Mahal.

David's: Paris beside me on a pew bathed together in the rainbow-colored light of La Rochelle's stained glass windows.

Maybe we'd give away everything we owned. Maybe stay right here in the house we built and love?

To know or not to know your journey's end date? That is the question. Love to hear what you think caregivers. If it's a dilemma you grapple with. Coping with "End of life planning?"

Loss came the answer. Devastating sense of loss. Weird after all my moaning how exhausting I found caregiving.

The phone rang yesterday. "This is George, your best friend."

I knew no George and was about to punch disconnect when he added, "Your husband stopped by at my stand at the Albuquerque Parkinson's Conference last week requesting information on pre-paid cremation."

So many stands, so many leaflets touting different information, the day's talks pushing alternative therapies of all the must dos we could-should be doing, the conference left me depressed if I am honest.

It wasn't the sight of so many gimped up people and their captive gaolers that punctured my spirit, no — it was the word *hope*.

"Never give up hope." The keynote speaker dunked the word *hope* to the audience. *Dunked* a new word for me, I pitched it to a corner of my mind.

The key-note speaker, star basketball athlete Brian Grant, introduced a video of him dunking ball after ball. Six foot nine, Rasta hair, a startlingly beautiful face, and perfectly proportioned body, he held the mike.

A flash of light caught my eye. The shifting sparkle of the diamonds framing his wristwatch jiggled, thrown by his tremor. A vice-grip of realization cramped my insides.

"This gorgeous chunk of humaity suffers from PD" I whispered to David. "So young." Was it all the more cruel because he was in his thirties, I questioned.

Early onset PD, Brian informed us. *I can play before a stadium of tens of thousands no problem, but you lot, an audience of fellow sufferers and caregivers has me shaking like a leaf."* He paused laughing and plunged his tremoring hand deep into his pocket.

Never give up hope. I never thought I'd climb a mountain, he looked directly at us. *I and five other PD sufferers,* he used the acronym for Parkinson's, *conquered Mount St Helens last summer. Hell of a struggle but we all made it to the summit.*

His saying *don't give up* is when I realized hope is exactly what I have surrendered. No cure, the caterpillar-like disease relentlessly biting chunks from David's and my lives. That was a day I was stuck. Depressed. Convinced we'd never to morph to butterflies.

You never asked for this, caregivers, the speaker continued.

Turning to us, the audience, he asked, *Any caregivers out there? Put your hands up. Thank you,* he said. *Thank you,* he repeated adding *you never asked for Parkinson's to be in your life, but everyone of you is suffering from Parkinson's too. You were never asked to give up your lives to caregiving, but you did. Thank you, I thank every one of you.*

It was then I started to cry. David apart, it was the first time I felt truly acknowledged, the first time anyone directly beamed deep gratitude from their heart.

Wearing hope's face mask when my insides are dust is hard. Hope is my only staff. Hope is what buoys me afloat. If hope slips away, what then...

... those days I find him slumped hollow-eyed a sand-dried carcass like the Red-tailed Hawk remains we came upon together walking barefoot in White Sands National Monument... those days like today when he sits slumped at breakfast one cheek hard pressed to the table, left arm hanging from the chair, fingers reaching the floor — beneath his cheek, a flattened muffin...

. ... those days I sink into the fathomless waters of the Blue Hole, wonder how long can I cope with him at home, those days I cry, "Help me make it through today."

*   *   *

"You realize he'll have to go into a home one day."

She, of all people, his sister, a geriatric nurse — is she nuts? Could a tortoise gouged from his shell keep living? Could David? Only if and when, like the poor buggers incapacitated, too aged, too financially strapped with no-one, then I suppose, social services would insist he be taken into care. Bodily bundle him away.

But today David is ON enough to insist, "I'm begging you to see to it, Liz. Don't let them invade my right to stay."

"You realize he'll have to go into a home, one day." His sister and her nurse-friend reiterated.

"He can just as well be a vegetable here in his own chair, if that's what he becomes." I countered frostily. "Paying for home care costs the same as a facility. I'll never let him die alone in some awful institution. NEVER."

Affirmed in love, occasionally repented in exhaustion, those days a scream rips, "I can't go on. I can't." I do and can of course. The same way I dragged from bed fevered and weak to tend my children many years ago.

"Better to die than come to that — go into a home." My husband had sworn. "I'll do away with myself."

A doctor — he surely squirreled a stash of knockout pills in a place only he knew. Don't tell. Don't ask. I never have.

I didn't sleep well that night for a nightmare of my David crumpled lopsided in a cage. Me passing spiked carrots and bananas to him through the bars. Me dragged away in handcuffs charged with murder. Last sight of him, an abandoned family pet in the pound, the pleading in his eyes.

I woke with the image nailed to my visual cortex.

"I love you so much," Planting kisses on his head while handing him a breakfast cereal bowl, I guide a spoon into his fumbling fingers, my face averted.

Are you plagued by nightmares, caregivers? It's hard remembering they are not real. It's hard keeping strong.

"Don't crumble," I tell myself. "We have lots of normal moments to remember."

Like the many times David eats a meal without me having to spoon-feed him. Like the evenings spent quietly together in the back yard drinking up the Indian Summer sun watching the peach tree shred her golden leaves. I fall for it, every time… we are a married couple again living with hope. Normal.

You couldn't be more correct that the nondisabled and their friends and family don't understand the joy of a day where everything seems normal. One of the things I learned from caregiving and now from working with people with Parkinsons is gratitude for every good moment. ~K J

13. disabled... daft... demented?

Disabled? Daft? Demented? Which is he?

Until last week's Cognitive test at the Movement Disorder Clinic in Phoenix, I insisted my husband David, was disabled not daft. But now the test results have declared him officially DEMENTED, I don't know what to think.

"He's crossed the line from DEMENTIA to DEMENTED," the neurologist peered at us from across his desk perhaps expecting us to cry hearing the diagnosis spoken out loud.

But to have it proved my sweetie-pie was DAFT, to hear the doctor state he was demented stunned me to silence.

David sat impassive un-fazed by the pronouncement. I suppressed a smile. OK, temporarily daft I could accept.

True, David often appeared mentally challenged when he switched off, flopped sideways unable to speak a word. But what of the many times his recall of names and places were better than mine, and his communication skills, speech and thoughts flowed grammatically correct. What of the fluent conversations we frequently shared?

Demented indeed — no absolutely not. I know the brilliant man I married lurks today cozy inside his shell.

Only last Sunday I overheard David chatting to his best friend correctly using the word specificity discussing the pros and cons of a particular seizure drug.

Only last month, when a distressed friend of mine broke down not knowing what to do about her teenage son's sudden raving in a psychotic episode. "Talk to David." I suggested and left them closeted together.

"David was fully on for the whole hour," she related later. "… and gave me the most helpful and perfect advice."

Made the demented diagnosis laughable really. Call it denial, resistance to me facing the truth, David's intelligence shone too often to accept the test's damming results. After all there were reasons to explain his low score.

A hole in his skull, for one thing. Caused when his mother tumbled down a flight of stairs with David clutched in her arms. He was two. The fall knocked out the spatial lobe of David's brain — a section of IQ tests that forever scored ZERO.

So he couldn't draw a clock face, or copy a shape? So what he flunked those tests? Brain damage explained the low overall numbers. After all, I excused, before PD, Stanford once classified him GENIUS.

STUPID, DAFT, DEMENTED different spins of one coin. Parkinson's dementia pops in, pops out. David too. The turtle image came to me–a turtle's rise and sinking to and from the water's surface.

"Today's date? The town we're visiting?" Easy.

Recalling details of a story, lists of objects, a series of numbers — not so easy.

Perhaps blanking out the incoming President's name was David's protest. A defiant gesture of rejection of the new Commander-in-Chief's twitter-mad Administration.

Guess what the Movement Disorder clinic discovered from the read-out of the ambulatory EEG hat? David's left temporal brain lobe was in and out of constant seizures, while the right lobe remained normal.

HURRAH. Seizures could be dealt with. We had a reason for David's unresponsive switched off episodes.

I swallow ashamed of the times I've yelled when my poor husband froze and I dragged at his walker, "This way. Mind where you're going. Lift your feet... " On and on.

"If you can't use your eyes, use your G'... dam brain." My shouting sticks in the walls.

He was seizuring – of course David couldn't move. Right himself in his chair or lift his cheek from the table. Of course he was unable to speak. Whatever the test showed, I knew he was no simpleton.

I shook my head. Why hadn't his local neurologist researched a reason for David's increasingly frequent off episodes when I'd asked her over and over again?

ACCEPT IT–"Freezing is just part of Parkinson's." Was the answer given. "... and anyway Ambulatory EEG is not covered by Medicare in this state."

DENIED–our request for further testing..

IGNORED–the danger of David falling, knocking himself out, fracturing a leg, his ribs, The frightening impact freezing has on our lives.

Like the moment three years back, de-planing in Frankfurt, the horror of the air stewards as he stiffened immobile, eyes glued shut, blocking the gangway; like the time in the Jacuzzi after warm water exercise class. The instructor wanted to call the ER and it took three men to haul him from the water and into a wheelchair.

No. No. No, you doctors out there who dismiss a symptom described by their patient or caregiver, NO it is not acceptable to fob us off with platitudes.

BE PRO-ACTIVE is the lesson. Don't let up.

INSIST on an informed answer. If you don't get one, Caregivers, LOOK ELSEWHERE. Another state if necessary.

Makes sense doesn't it to find out what is going on in the brain? Thanks to a presentation to our local Parkinson's support Group, we found the Neurologist who suggested mapping David's brainwaves.

I'm surprised how much I'm more relaxed, gentle towards David even, now I understand David's not being obstinate when he does not respond. Seizures are the culprits not him.

DEMENTED- despite the finding, people speaking for David drives me nuts.

"What would HE like?" Pencil and pad poised to take our order the waitress looks at me not him.

I do speak for him when it is obvious David cannot respond. I barrage him with forced alternatives — yes/no questions — wait for his nod, headshake to order his menu choice.

"Lasagna? Shepherd's Pie? Caesar salad?"

To my mind, addressing him directly is only polite. Is showing respect too much to ask? I have a friend who says, yes.

Yes, it is too much to expect of people, busy wait staff for example; too much to expect others to give him a chance to answer before turning to me and talking over him.

She, my friend, says it is not a stranger's business to deal with his slowness — to have them wait awkwardly while David gathers his thoughts. Forms a reply.

"That's your job, not theirs," she tries to convince me. "Face it. When David acts demented, he is. It's downright rude of you to put a stranger in an uncomfortable position. David too."

Oooh, I don't quite like what she says. It gives me pause. Something to mull over before taking him out to a restaurant again.

I ask you caregivers, *do you agree?*

I like our Family Practioner. I'm grateful he speaks to David directly. Asks the usual how-are-you-what's-going-on questions. Waits patiently wondering if David heard the question. David sits GONE no answer forthcoming. I am forced to ask, "David would you like me to answer for you?" and when David nods, I rattle on speaking for him.

Slow brainwaves are a part of his Parkinson's picture, we've learned from the EEG.

That is all I ask — the chance to speak for himself before turning to me. Surely the difference between disabled and daft is obvious without carrying a banner?

Not a bad idea in one respect. Perhaps he should wear a T-shirt plastered with I'M NOT AN IDIOT. IT'S PARKINSON'S.

Encountering someone normal looking who gives a sudden lurch, acts clumsy or plain odd is scary I now realize.

David's walker proclaims, HEY, I'M DISABLED. Walking sticks, wheelchairs, a blind friend's dark glasses and white stick, my deaf son's cochlear gadget stuck to the side of his head, an artificial limb...

Guess what, Caregivers, visibility helps a stranger understand a person is disabled.

I discovered this last week in Phoenix during a three-day, round the clock brain test requiring him to sleep, eat, and walk with his head bandaged like a wounded soldier. Down his back a trail of colored wires attached to a battery pack labeling him disabled.

"Let me help you." Doors opened and were held till we had passed. "Would he be more comfortable in a chair with arms?" Where I imagined stares and awkwardness driving us to hole up in our motel room, strangers smiled empathetic.

Question: Am i daft because i do daft things too? Lose keys... Squirrel away special chocolate treats never to find them for months... Search for my reading glasses to discover them on my nose...

Does being forgetful make me daft? Or acting without thinking? Plunging into a Guatemalan lake before checking, for example.

Discovering too late the jetty from which I jumped was the alligators' favorite spot to cool off. Brrr. I shiver… sharp teeth… ripped flesh… my stupidity.

Perhaps it is me who is daft or *Doolally Tap* as my father used to say — a village in India where mentally disturbed British soldiers were treated.

I often talk to myself now. Worry I'm losing it.

Example: last week when I bundled David to the airport on the wrong day and we missed the flight. Then yesterday. Engrossed, tap-tapping words on this computer I forgot David's pills, not only to count them but to give them.

More often now, I obliterate the present… emails, kitchen chores, phone calls — you know — normal stuff — and, well, plain forget.

"Just stress," I excuse myself. "I'm operating on auto-pilot, that's all."

"Remember," I tell myself, "… remember to remind David to remind me to… Now what the devil was it I had to remember to do?"

> I think it's very good that you're writing these blogs, both for yourself and for readers who, like me, haven't had to learn these particular lessons yet. I share your anger against the arrogance and officiousness of the nurses, physical therapists etc. with whom you're contending, and am indignant along with you. ~DdV

February, 4, 2017

14. up up and away...

Up. Up and away... not in a balloon, though that would be fun, but in a chair lift scaling a precipitous mountain in the French Alps. Lake Benit lay hidden in a crater out of reach to David and me. We'd called ahead to find out if the chair lift would take somebody so handicapped.

"Mais oui. We stop the lift, help him on, stop it again to help him off... et voila."

I pictured the frenchness of his shrug. Imagined the incredulous *are-you-mad-you-didn't* exclamations of our friends back in the litigation-fearing States; the disclaimer forms we'd be forced to sign should the lift operators even agree to allow him on.

This happened just two summers back when David's balance often tipped him to the ground and he could no longer hold his body upright. Legs dangling swinging above the pines, clutching the safety bar across holding us in the chair we made it to the summit, our children and grandchildren encouraging. The only person fussing — me.

Oooo. I shiver — the clang and judder of the chairlift bumping along the wire.

The scary ride was worth it — the picnic and view — a dream. Leaving David propped happy in a folding chair among the crocus and blue gentian, we scattered to explore. Shame I didn't have my camera ready when I returned, captured the scene, David hunkered in his chair encircled by a herd of curious cows.

It seems David attracts them. Once in Costa Rica returning from his walk, I met David, sheepish, behind him a string of maybe eleven cows plodding in his footsteps along the black sand beach.

Memories such as these are what support me when I sink depressed. Uplift me and remind me, Parkinson's or no, we can and still do have fun.

What I am saying, is don't hold back. Be bold. Defy the damnable disease. I'm surprised how much David is still keen to do with gentle prodding.

If I have anything to offer, Caregivers, I'd say jump at every chance to take a flying leap at all the wild things you've dreamed of doing while you can.

Ride that air balloon, paraglide the air currents beside the ravens riding tandem... Learn a new language? Why ever not. Walk the treadmill? Don't listen to fuddy-duddies who insist it's too dangerous, just make sure somebody is with him. Compete in the Senior Olympics? Hell yes. Go for it and DO.

David and I took up ping-pong just a couple of months ago. Fearless, at first David staggered backwards after every ball and sometimes fell, but now? He's become a tiger. Zip, zip, his improved balance, hand:eye:mind coordination the ball skims the net.

"I'd like to sign up for the Chi Center's Qigong Course," David surprised me last week. So we did. Lasted the full eight hours.

"I'd like to try medical marijuana," he declared a year ago. Helped a little but not enough to renew his card.

Fly? Why not? "If he can sit in a chair watching TV for hours, then why not in a plane?"

We ordered wheelchair assistance at the airports, found people to rent our house and took off.

Up, up and away we went…

a bamboo palapa in the trees above the beach in Mexico… snakes and rain in Belize… the ruins of Tikal in the Guatemalan jungle… hot springs and volcanoes in Chile… summers in Spain, Italy, Scotland, France… ten days in a rubber dingy riding through the Grand Canyon rapids…

We crammed our lives.

"Sri Lanka was the best of all," David said one day thumbing through an album and laughing at the image of himself wielding a machete attempting to hack open a coconut and remembering how his sarong slipped, leaving him starkers.

Turning a page, topless, I walk again the black sands on the isolated beach beyond the ginger plants and lemon grasses around our shack. Call songs of love to the waves.

Could fourteen years have passed since Kerala?

"Damn weird place to honeymoon," the family remarked when I told them we were off to an Ayurveda Nursing Home in India for a month's treatment."

Our quarters were a sand-floored hut, our bathroom open to the air with a resident scorpion in the basin, and bed with a coconut-coir filled mattress. We were in heaven. David checked in with a fading voice, and head constantly moving.

Twenty-eight days later checked out with a strong voice and head no longer jiggling. Exhausted, oiled, pummeled, clear-skinned and healthy, "It took six weeks on a beach recovering," we jest.

This winter we're off to Puerto Vallarta for two weeks. Vacation and dental work combined same as every year for the past seven. Cheaper dentist, the savings make our holiday free — well, almost.

This year I'm nervous managing David on my own so a good friend will share our space. Boost my confidence. Help me.

"Hey, hurry, hurry, David, look, a double rainbow. Let's sit on the porch and watch," I exclaim, shuffling him through the door.

It is too easy for the two of us to slump feet up, stare at nothing, and slide into the ether. You too, I suspect caregivers, if you're as tired as I am.

Parkinson's disease weighs so heavy sometimes. Squashes me flat. David's shell sits keeled to one side unresponsive. No cajoling hauls him to the present. Would he ever return?

I pretend he isn't there. Re-focus on *Lilies*, a British film I'm half watching. Fight back tears, forgetting we were once a regular couple that met and fell in love at our village rodeo 35 years ago... our courtship of eighteen years.

"Remember when... " I coax myself. Drop my caregiver mantle. Revived by memories. Happy ones... his joke as we signed the Marriage License, "I don't know what the hurry is."

My husband, my David, my best friend, floats into a world beyond my reach.

I turn my head and see not the wrecked human he now is, but the sensitive, gentle being who first introduced me to the heavy yellow orb releasing slowly from the mesa, flooding the Galisteo basin with a moonrise so bright we saw each rock and juniper tree. I'd noticed no such beauty in suburban England. Barely witnessed a sunset through her grey pall.

It came to me then: proportionally speaking these down years are but a small toll to pay for the thirty years of good. I have enough memories tucked into my brain to see me through.

Change the prescription of your glasses, I once heard an Indian Spiritual Master teach.

I bought a pair of rose-tinted glasses. Keep them on my puja, altar, as a reminder to see the world in a different way. After all isn't there a silver lining in everything? Difficult to think *what* sometimes. Well... his Parkinson's, my caregiver role has brought us closer, that's certain.

Worked my character over too—most likely for the better.

Parkinson's? Yes, the disease has taught me to see the less abled in a kinder light, discover what matters in our lives. Educated us in subjects we'd never heard of before P.D.

Without David I'd be rattling alone in an empty nest wanting him back…

"Give us a year together, God," I prayed before we got married. "Please don't let Parkinson's Disease take him from me just yet."

So far we've clocked fourteen years.

How I feel for you and the adjustment you are going through as caregiving morphs into a 24-hour grind Of course you're not a failure. The two of you are together thanks to your strength and love. I liken myself to any human finding themselved imprisoned for life. I have a Choice·Fight what can't be changed and go nuts· or by blinkering the past and seeing only the present, discover, if not happiness at least a little contentment. If it's any encouragement I can see from the softening of tone between blog number 1 and the later ones, this past year has changed me. I think because I've fully accepted caregiving is my new norm.   ~ Liz.

15. humble Pie

Humble Pie — yum. Tastes surprisingly good. Took a little while… months in fact… to take that first bite and step foot inside our local Senior Center. We entered its door only to vote and collect our trash passes before that.

Now I have, I can't imagine why I skirted the place as if by entering I might catch some dreaded disease. Wrinkles? Grey hair perhaps? Was I that vain I refused to admit David and I fit right in with its aged population? Or that by admitting to being *one of them* I was taking some sort of dangerous first step into quicksand from which I'd never break free?

"Mirror, mirror on the wall… tell me, please, I'm not the oldest looking of them all." Peering at my reflection I plucked a grey hair from my head. Saw only the smooth British complexion of my long forgotten youth, ignoring my age-spotted cheeks and wrinkles.

Admit my age? No way. I've always had a problem confessing how old I am.

"Age is a number and mine is unlisted." I'd fob off anyone rude enough to ask.

Turning fifty I never told a soul preferring to forgo the milestone celebration.

Me? Confess I was eligible for the AARP 10% discount offered by motels? No way. I paid the full rate. How snooty was that?

Ridiculous looking back. An age-snob, I confess. After all who the hell cared? Only me. Vain person I was and hope am no longer.

Before I turned eleven I felt more like a parcel than a child. One to be picked up and dropped wherever adults chose. Removed from my mother, half-sister and Ayah in India... dumped with an abusive caretaker... shipped to England and a Children's Home, before finally being given haven in the English countryside safe from a world beyond our driveway.

No fault of mine, I had no real opportunity to mix with regular folk closeted as I was with loving guardians on their farm in Gloucestershire.

If I ever was standoffish, it was because in the dreamworld where I lived inside my head, I preferred to clamber fences and wander the fields, hide in my beech tree, and venture on painting excursions with my guardian rather than playing with strange children.

It's not that I didn't want to be part of a group because I did. Since childhood I envied groups' noisy mixing, yearned to belong in somebody's circle — anybody's. The Children's Home didn't count. There, as one of the herd I avoided being singled out for punishment.

Not until I left home did I discover people — so many nationalities, so many variations, personalities, ways of thinking, being...

Then came David. Then came Parkinson's. Then came me-his care-partner. I found myself doing things I never dreamed of.

Face-wiping, foot-shoving toes into slippers, legs through trousers... I watched his dignity compromised by helplessness: the peaceful balance of our home disintegrate into a chaos of broken objects, stained floors tiles, and soiled furnishings.

Pictures tilt crooked, clocks stand frozen, newspaper and magazines pile unread and, well, as for the kitchen, I can barely fight my way in.

I love order, the careful placement of a vase, a sculpture or a treasured pebble. Wine sparkling in fine crystal, the feel of my favorite coffee mug, sitting down to a set table, used to give me pleasure.

Still would if… Well, anything goes now.

During one of those getting-to-know-the-other talks when David and I were first together. "If we are ever incapacitated, David, let's never, never be the other's caregiver. Better to hire a nurse whatever it costs. I'd be a rotten nurse and just don't have it in me. What's more it would ruin our relationship." I clearly remember saying. Vehement.

What do they say… *never say never?*

Should I have listened, I tell myself ruefully because our relationship has changed and not, dare I admit it, entirely for the better? I stare at David's false teeth in my hand.

"These are your uppers David. Turn the damn things other side up No the other way round, dammit."

Ever since seeing my father's gnashers smiling in a glass of murky water, I'd sworn, "No false teeth for me. Never ever… "

Yes, caregiving is a leveler. No question about it. What I'm struggling to say is my caregiver role has made me more accepting, more empathetic. Humbled me in fact.

I am a human, bound by rules and convention. A bird is just one of the flock and instinctively does what birds do. I wish my life was as easy. That I could just loosen up. I'm working on it — slowly letting go the ironclad rules with which I've bound myself. Appearances for instance. Comfort over convention is at last a choice.

Favorite belts and smart waist-banded trousers hang neglected in the closet. Pull-on-pull-off zipper-less, button-less jogging pants, make for easier dressing, less toilet accidents and give David more autonomy. Cozy too. Until David looks like a hobo, David's stubble no longer bothers me. We're often too whacked out to shower daily.

As for me — I can't wait to remove my bra and snuggle into my slops come evenings. Unimaginable now — as a teen in my guardians' home, wearing trousers to the dinner table was forbidden.

About a year ago I was waiting for the trash permit at our Senior

Center, when the lively babble from the crowded tables in the room beyond attracted me to take a peek. Most of the *old folk* enjoying lunch didn't look that old. Hmm.

Leaving I paused at the notice board — chair yoga, chair-aerobics, strengthening and stretch classes, pottery, painting, indoor gardening — so many classes FREE and a lifetime's membership for just $4. Wow, couldn't beat that.

Parkinson's literature lays great store by exercise. Yes, the Chair Strengthening class would do David good.

"I suppose I could take the class too having driven him all this way," I conceded. "Though I'm way too fit and young for this."

Reluctantly I raised my knees from the chair and joined the forty pairs of waving arms and legs. But I envied them, their confidence. How they flung themselves into every activity.

Looking over, a wheelchair-bound woman lifted the stump of her amputated leg following as best she could. What guts. I was ashamed of my arrogance.

David is brave too. I watch the effort it takes to lift his foot off the floor. Attempt ankle rotation. He is engrossed. Shames me into giving my best.

We check the menu, sign up for lunch a couple of days a week nowadays. No shopping, food prep, no clean-up. Food not bad either. If she only knew what she's missing....

I laugh remembering a friend's 90 year-old mother. "What eat with all those *old grey hairs* — Never."

I think of the stories I've heard, of lives in Burma, Malaysia, Kuwait and Alaska, the people I've met over lunch at the Senior Center... a Brit born in India, a man from the Peace Corps in Haiti, the visitor in his Pushtun woolen hat from Medicin Frontier, who worked with the Afridi and other tribal groups.

Perhaps I should ask each their story. I see the gimped up differently now I've put on these rose-tinted specs. Shifted perspective.

"Hello," I encourage. Smile at Norman's kindly care, the gentle way he guides his disabled wife to her chair, places cutlery in her hand. Wipes food from her chin. Wish I had his patience.

"You should join the Parkinson's support group," a girlfriend encouraged when I complained I was at my wits end.

"Yeah. Yeah. It's just one more thing on the calendar. One day... " I lied. Listening to other peoples moaning was the last thing I needed.

Foolish me. Knowledge is Power goes the aphorism. And it's true. Thanks to the information gleaned from our local Parkinson's Support Group, I am better armed to understand and question treatments, medications and new research.

PARKINSON'S ACTION is group's new name. Active they are. Without them and their expert speakers David and I would never have heard of NOH, never heard of an ambulatory EEG, gone to Arizona's Movement Disorder Clinic, learned of a bacterial Parkinson's brain-gut connection, discovered Rock Steady Boxing, the Thera-cycle and other alternative approaches to wellness.

Teachy-preachy, or not Caregivers, I beg you don't put off finding or forming a support group as late as we did. Should have done it years ago.

Another *should-have* —

Months back, years perhaps, I should have combed every government and private source for help. Instead I waited. Chanted the *I-don't-deserve-it, I-don't-need-charity* platitudes refusing to admit my desperate need. Yes, i do need help. Surprise.

When I finally asked for help, Senior Social Services offered some. Twice weekly a man drives twenty-five miles to shower and shave David to take him places. Gives me a little respite. He and David are friends now.

Don't know what my problem has been with receiving help. After all should someone give me a gift voucher to a swank restaurant, I say *cheers* and *thanks*.

"Help offered is a gift. So bite your lip and accept what you're offered with grace," I admonish myself.

It took a homeless man panhandling at the road junction to teach me to ask for help.

"I NEED HELP please." His cardboard sign pleaded. Me too I realized as I handed him a dollar bill. Saw his gratitude.

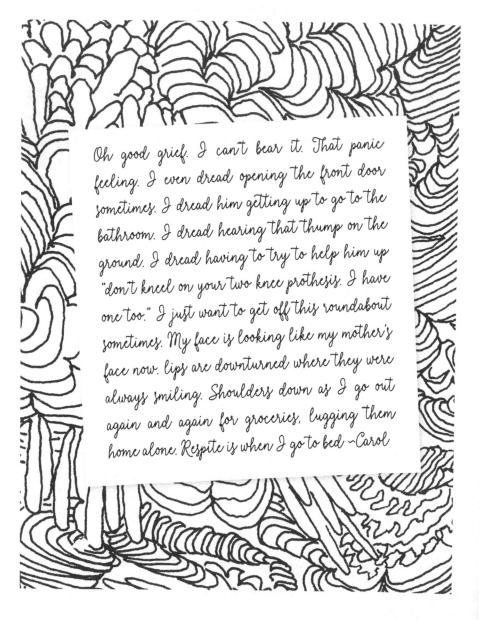

Oh good grief. I can't bear it. That panic feeling. I even dread opening the front door sometimes. I dread him getting up to go to the bathroom. I dread hearing that thump on the ground. I dread having to try to help him up "don't kneel on your two knee prothesis. I have one too." I just want to get off this roundabout sometimes. My face is looking like my mother's face now. lips are downturned where they were always smiling. Shoulders down as I go out again and again for groceries. lugging them home alone. Respite is when I go to bed ~Carol

February 18, 2017

16. what do i have to complain about?

Moan, moan, moan. *YOU'RE NOT ALONE,* friends soothe. It doesn't help, you know — telling me. I know friends mean well offering pop-in help and I am grateful, truly, but fact is David and I are adrift alone in a sea of day to day survival.

Try a caregiver's life for twenty-four hours and then tell me. Try coping on three or four hours sleep. *Go to bed earlier.* I imagine you advising. But that's impossible don't you see. I can't till David's safely tucked up.

"Ready? Ready yet, David? Teeth? Clothes off? Slippers? Washed? Please hurry, I'm dropping."

Familiar isn't it Caregivers, functioning asleep on our feet?

My sleep cycle now broken by activity, I lie in bed for hours counting sheep? — forget those woolly bundles jumping gates, tomorrow's to-dos are what I'm counting. I try stars next, get caught up wandering the universe, and following moving lights across the heavens — could one be a UFO?

One a.m. "Blast," I swear, "it's now nearly two." I'm clock watching.

Sleep aids? No luck with teas or pills. CBD, high-free cannabis oil? Tomorrow I must sign on and get some. I imagine driving the twisting road to Colorado… snooze deeply. Morning comes two seconds after my eyelids close it seems.

"What time is it?" David asks mid dream before first light, before

I'm ready to be a giver of care.

"Too early, David." I roll away. Remembering he needs me, I roll back to see David standing by my pillow. A pair of scissors dangles in his hand.

Chore number one of the day: snip off wet security underwear. Change him into dry ones.

"Too early David," I growl after I've made him comfortable. "Go back to bed." Within a second snoring rattles from his room. "Lucky bugger," I fume. Try reading. Try sips of hot tea. Give up. Get up.

"Terrible night. Just couldn't fall asleep," I glower over breakfast. "Watch out I'll be a crabby bitch all day."

Complaining won't change a thing I realize. I'm venting that's all. And I know my life isn't ALL toil and grind and we still have heaps of fun.

Take today's swim class peddling our exercise noodles. Legs pumping, arms waving, laughing, being silly, David and I narrowly missing one another — circus performers on unicycles.

Take the lecture we attended, the film that held us spellbound, or the birthday party of a friend — the warm snuggle we share if I've hopped into his bed.

Bed, now there's a word to make me grateful.

BED. I'm pulled back to the night drive through Mumbai from the airport over a dozen years ago. Rows of crates line the pavement. Four-tiered accommodation for the homeless: on top of the crate, inside the crate, a sheet of cardboard on the sidewalk, then the least desirable and by far the worst — children even — curled on the hard pavement, legs sticking into the traffic.

Yes, life could be WORSE. David and I have no idea how much worse... Parkinson's or no, with more blessings than fingers to count them, we are so very lucky.

Today David surprised me — got almost dressed without my help.

Small achievement, you may judge, but I saw it as a gift.

Our home's paid for, we have each other, and a mountain view whose white peaks sing the horizon. We have enough money to choose what and when we want to eat, what clothes to wear, and what to do with our time — luxury enough to balance the Parkinson's horribles.

If a handful of earth and sky hold no emptiness as Hafiz declares, I have more riches than I can count.

"What's more," I scold myself. "I have the freedom of choice,"

Location, job, socio-economic status, life has swung me up, down and turned direction often. Making the switch from speech therapy to sculpture, sculpture to writing came easy. Working in a calm office with music playing, beat pounding heavy bags of clay.

Giving up time to devote to David's care — not so easy. Words, thoughts pile heaped unwritten in my mind.

The computer keys stand lifeless, beckon me to sneak away and get tapping. But hey…

After all what's more important — my beloved husband's wellbeing or chasing some elusive fame by finishing my book about Spain, or the sequel to *Poet Under A Soldier's Hat* (the book I wrote illustrating one hundred years of Colonial Rule in India through the personal stories of one family — mine as it happens.)

The answer: David. No question. He, me, us, our karma together — we're what matters. Parkinson's, my caregiver role, life's circumstance — are what has been dished to us this lifetime round.

"Better get used to it baby, this is what's is," I counsel myself. Nice concept. No quite so easy to carry out. I am still struggling deciding what part of me to chop. Forget should. Forget duty. Forget if only…

"This is the life you've been given by God. Live it fully." Reads one of two quotes I keep on my puja. The second reads, "Whatever you do let it come from a place of love."

I stand back up, my direction clear. Shared joys. Simple pleasures — those I'll dwell on. Mini hikes, desert drives and bird watching from our living room.

Yes, I have to pack and load David's heavy walker into the car for expeditions. Yes, I have to help him on with his shoes, coat, scarf and hat.

Remember pills, drinking water, sunglasses and hiking poles, but oh the exhilaration of getting out freed from our grotty world of daily coffee spills and trampled macaroni beneath his chair, to walk a leaf-strewn mountain path of brilliant yellow.

One example.

"Let's drive to Aspen Meadows," David suggested last fall.

"How beautiful was that?" We sighed back home.

Life lessons are all about me when I'm tuned to reach for my rose-tinted specs — see things differently. Even surveillance cameras, would you believe?

Picture seven people, age range five to seventy-five. Returning home by car after a glorious week on the Mediterranean.

We'd just turned onto the Grenoble autoroute from Voiron when the engine died. Panic — we'll all be killed. No way could David jump the fence to avoid the frantic shoal of speeding holiday traffic. Pulling on the obligatory green breakdown jackets and setting warning triangles back and front, our son and daughter-in-law flapped orange jackets fearful we'd all be mown down.

Before we could phone for help an orange rescue vehicle trundled into view, behind it a tow-truck. A surveillance camera spotting the breakdown automatically dispatched a rescue crew — hoisted us away.

"A welcome intrusion," I now describe those big brother eyes — those invasive spies I'd so derided.

No special dinner, no dozen red roses, February the fourteenth,

David opened his card.

"Will you be my Valentine?" The words crooned.

"Yes," he said. "Will you be mine?"

"Yes," I answered.

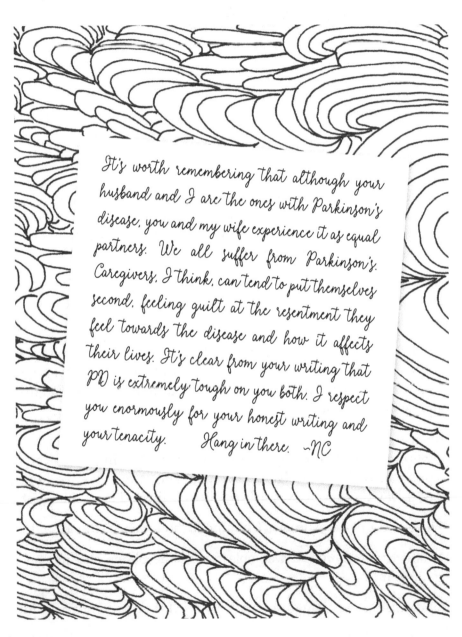

It's worth remembering that although your husband and I are the ones with Parkinson's disease, you and my wife experience it as equal partners. We all suffer from Parkinson's. Caregivers, I think, can tend to put themselves second, feeling guilt at the resentment they feel towards the disease and how it affects their lives. It's clear from your writing that PD is extremely tough on you both. I respect you enormously for your honest writing and your tenacity. Hang in there. ~NC

February 25, 2017

17. come back tooth fairy

Here we are again in Puerto Vallarta, Mexico for our annual visit to the dentist. Set me thinking.

The perfect excuse for a holiday, we have added dental tourism to our list of to-dos. After reading about our experience, dental tourism might be worth considering Caregivers, if like us, you are strapped for cash and have no insurance.

"It's time we paid a visit to the dentist," we sigh come February when winter winds howl their worst. "Oh dear," we wink. "We'll have to fly to P.V."

David's tremor was under control when we took our first dental trip. Though balance problems, the worst of his symptoms back then, had him lurching and crashing about like a drunk. Fatigue often wiped him out. And he was fast becoming toothless.

About eight or seven years ago David's smile revealed small brown points in a gappy mouth. I could show you a frightening photograph to prove it. With just twelve stubs remaining something had to be done if David wasn't to waste away, forever limited to a liquid diet.

"I'll get a couple of estimates from the orthodontists," David said.

He still drove then and was able to use the phone and manage by himself.

But dentists are no laughing matter — until they present you with their bill that is. A Picasso canvas doesn't fetch so much per inch as teeth framed alluringly in gums. Returning from the consultations David announced,

"$50,000 for ten implants.... um... ," he hesitated seeing my jaw slacken and my eyes jam wide, "... err... without crowns or X-rays, and then I'll need... "

I didn't let him finish. I leapt to my feet,

"Unreal. Are they barking mad? Sell or re-mortgage our home, is that what the bastards want? You'll have to chew with what you've got, have the lot pulled out... better off wearing false plates ... or a set of wooden teeth like George Washington. We could buy a B.M.W. with that."

My face reddened, scorched the estimate in his hand. "Outrageous. The greed... "

"But whatever to do?" David shook his head. "I have to eat."

"Dental Tourism. That's the answer. I've read about it somewhere."

My google research revealed a host of choices, Thailand, Bulgaria, Costa Rica, India and Mexico, the list stretched long.

We settled on the nearest, Mexico, and an ocean resort on the 'holiday package deal' route. We pored over websites, judging the clinics by their specialties and their command of English. E-mails buzzed through cyberspace. We asked around.

Nearest was best we both agreed and settled on Puerto Vallarta a long established wintering-hole of American and Canadian Snowbirds, and retirees owning second homes.

"Wealthy people don't put up with second-rate dentistry. They'll be sure of finding a P.V. dentist as good as theirs back home," we argued. We were right.

"Guess what? For the $$$ we'll save we'll get free holiday as well."

We burrowed in the storage boxes in our shed, packed our bags with light summer clothes, swimming togs, sun-screen, and boogie board, waved the snow-threatening sky goodbye and headed for the sun and salty sea.

Living in the high, mountain desert of New Mexico as we did, just the thought of humidity and warmth, our desiccated skin hydrated.

The hotel hugged a golden stretch of sand; the restaurant over-looked the ocean; our room vibrated with the tide's lullaby. A salt-rimmed glass of margarita in our hand, Happy Hour was happy hour every hour, everyday except those spent at the dentist.

First appointment. David's and my guarded expression advertised our fears. A Canadian in the dentist's waiting room started chatting.

"You've come to the best dentist in all of Mexico," he assured us. "My wife and I come every year."

The sunlit waiting room gleamed, polished. A sculptured basin in the restroom ran hot and cold. The toilet flushed. The dental assistants' matching uniforms rustled comfortingly crisp. Digital computer screens stood by every chair.

One dentist for root canals, one for extractions and a third for gum surgery I noted. So far so good. I relaxed, made an appointment for myself. A pillow beneath my head, supine in the dental chair, Vaseline on my lips, but for the brief sting as of a bee, I floated, painless from beneath my shades, as soft hands probed, drilled and did what dentists do. David didn't get off so easily, poor fellow.

"I've discussed the best course of action with my colleagues," Dr. P. reassured. "At your age and with your Parkinson's' issues we don't think you should have to go through implant surgery," he advised David, "We suggest the less invasive, less expensive treatment of posts and crowns."

Spread over the following three weeks, David endured eight ap-pointments of several hours each.

"You doing OK? Like a ten-minute break?"

"Arrgh! Ha! Arrgh! Ha!" He grunted in response.

Finally his ordeal over, he flashed a photogenic smile sporting nineteen usable teeth.

"My handsome husband's back. You look great, darling. At last your photograph won't break the camera."

Time in the dental chair and the days consuming endless bowls of soup while our gums healed were but a small price to pay for our holiday.

The final visit arrived, squeezed into our last day. My husband smiled a Hollywood smile sporting nineteen gnashers.

In a month, once the gums have healed and shrunk to size, what a dreadful shame, would mean winging our way back to P.V. on an off-season package deal, for two more weeks in the sun.

"Poor us — Such hardship." Friend's eyes narrow, green when we tell them.

We knew we'd made the right decision to do our dental work in Mexico when one of David's temporary crowns flipped off its base due to his excessive flossing. A ten-minute visit to glue them back up here in the U.S. cost us the equivalent of half a complete crown down in Mexico. Or five dental cleanings with the dentist's inspections included.

David caught my eye, nibbled rabbit teeth behind the receptionist's back while she ran his credit card. We just made it outside before breaking into ironic laughter.

"Unbelievable, the GREED of them," we exploded.

Friends shy skeptical. Still do, though they pester us with questions. Mutter on about trust, workmanship, and getting shot...

"Dental tourism works for us," we flash our smiles, clack our teeth. "See?"

My job as David's caregiver has its perks. Playing guide on dental trips is one.

He emerged with a good looking smile of nineteen usable teeth.

18. Promises Promises

Promises, Promises.

Do you, like me cling to hope fellow Caregivers? Fall again and again for the fantasy that our loved-ones and lives are back to normal? Wishful thinking I suppose. Riding a magic carpet reinforces my purpose.

What gets me is the uncertainty, the never knowing if he, my David, is *in, out, on or off, above water or below.* From one minute to the next, poof, he can vanish. Or Cheshire-cat himself back. I can't tell you how many times I've fooled myself believing David's here beside me — my best friend and lover back once more.

"Hello David," I reach to grab him. Open my palm to a handful of fool's dust.

Take today for instance. Awake and alert after an appointment in town David suggested we lunch at a nearby Chinese café. He walked to the car unaided, strapped himself in, and exited towards the entrance by himself with no me push-pulling him to his feet — one hell of a deal, believe me.

Taking our seats, we ordered, and we sipped our hot and sour soup. I began to enjoy myself. So far, so good. Then the main dish arrived. His eyes sealed shut. I watched David's spoon lift upwards. His mouth opened. Chewed air.

"It's empty. Nothing on it." Harsh, my voice slid into his ear.

I piled a shrimp and a little rice onto his spoon and gripping his wrist guided his hand mouth-ward. As in the nursery tale when Sleeping Beauty's princess pricking her finger on the spinning wheel, David froze tilted to the left. Disappeared. I abandoned my chopsticks. My rice set to concrete in my gut.

"Sit up. We're in public," I hissed.

Coaxing, threatening, nothing roused him. "Oh no. What now?" I fretted. "How ever to get him up and out?"

Temptingly I pushed a fortune cookie between his fingers. Pah.

Something good is on its way.

Fat chance. I scrunched the slip into the plate's debris and signed the check. The man at the next table helped me get David to his feet.

"This is the last time, the very last, I swear I'll take him to a restaurant." Well... till the next time he suggests we eat out.

Why don't I listen to myself? Broke my word within the month. I can't believe I did it again. But I did, I dined with him in public.

Invited to a writers' awards banquet, I was a wee bit horrified when David firmly announced, "I'd like to come. Support you in case your name is called."

"Great," I answered before I could stop myself. Before pictures flashed of David keeled angled 90 degrees to the left, eyes closed and mute. Me, my poise crumbled guiding him and falling to the floor.

Previewing the evening I got myself in quite a tizzy. Because, and rightly so, with David by my side, attention revolves around him. AND it's impossible to have an uninterrupted conversation.

I looked forward to leaving behind my caregiver shoes for just one carefree evening. No appendages. Me alone, my own person free to schmooze swapping info and suchlike as an equal to fellow writers.

How to tell him no? Tell him, "Do you mind darling, I'd like this evening for myself." I didn't of course.

Couldn't bring myself to go back on my word. Hurt his feelings. Tell him I'd changed my mind and wanted — needed, even — to go to the event *alone* knowing that if I had, my food would have turned to mud.

"Anyway," I excused, "… too late to tell him for this year."

Next time if there is a next, I swear I will.

"How about I drive down to the venue, help him inside. I'll find a ta-ble and wait while you park?" David's sometime sitter volunteered.

I badly wanted to sit with… well, *interesting* people. Imagined the *oh-please-don't-sit-here* looks seeing us approach.

"Because nobody will want to sit with us," I whined.

No point denying having more than a hello-how-are-you two-way conversation with someone as disabled as David is so clearly — let's face it — IS too horribly difficult for most people to sustain. Me too.

Exceptions being the rule, that evening proved me wrong.

"Come join us," our table-mates welcomed pointing to the two vacant chairs. Lively conversations ping-ponged across the rubber chicken, over David's back and mingled with the wine.

The nightmarish angst I experienced before that banquet was my never-again lesson, my wake-up call to listen to myself.

"I promise, I promise to never again invite David to a fancy affair."

Embarrassments aside, I just don't have the strength in me to push-pull him upright, deal with spills, slobber and crashing cutlery. I get too damn stressed to have any fun.

Bored after six week's of home cooking, and plain lunches along-side other messy eaters at the Senior Center,

"I'd like to treat you to a decent meal out," David offered one day.

"That's lovely of you, darling, but eating out at posh restaurants is just not possible."

See, I am learning. It's the hardest thing isn't it caregivers — to admit defeat. Say no thanks, sorry, but *no can do*.

"What about the buffet at your club? We're still social members." I compromised.

Though David's tennis are long over, he clings to one of the last vestiges of the life he led before Parkinson's disease felled him.

All those retirees, David blends right in. White damask cloth, fire blazing, wine with the meal, friendly staff, there we can still play-act elegant.

Was I brave or foolhardy to take David to the movies alone? I'm still shaken from yesterday's outing.

Need to get this off my chest. Think maybe taking him alone will be the last time — *bloody well should be, okay? OKAY. I'll think about it* — ran the conversation in my head. But that was after...

I scurried David to the car and made our seats in time to see the kill-your cell phone message on the screen.

I couldn't decipher the accents for the first fifteen minutes. Then wished I hadn't for all the foul language understanding revealed.

"Do you want to leave, David?" I asked, hoping he would because the movie's sordid violence was nothing that interested me. But no, David insisted he'd like to watch the rest. Watch? Right — head back with his eyes tight closed — yes, some way to see.

I lost interest in the plot. Plotted a strategy how to ever get him up and out — justly as I was about to find out. Seated in the back row and unable to reach his armpits, Heave-hoeing, I hauled his frame upright by his coat collar and trundled him towards the exit.

Bad move. David turned facing back into the auditorium and froze where he stood imprisoning the exiting audience. Now what? Now what to do? I began to sweat. Wildly look around for help.

"Oh thank you. Yes, please," I said as the husband of the elderly couple jammed next to us waiting to leave each grabbed an arm and together the three of us push-pulled him from the doorway to the elevator.

Despite her own disability his wife brandished her cane insisting her husband help us to the car.

"That's it. Cross movie-going off our list. Can't and mustn't do that again," I muttered. "Not fair to him. Not fair to me. Not fair to strangers."

I'd better add another *do not* to my list. Movie-going.

Absolutely, I hear you exclaim. *What's taken you so long to get it?*

"What give up another one of our remaining treats?" I retort, defiant not wanting to accept the obvious.

Am I so feeble I cannot manage David single-handed? It's not that I'm set on movie going. Really. And in truth I'm not, what with Netflix' and Roku's endless selections to choose from.

Retiring my Lacrosse Stick I felt the same pang of loss, giving my tennis racquet to Goodwill, my piano to a family with young children, the realization high-heeled shoes were positively bone breakers at my age.

Yup. Reality can close a door or two. But, dare I spout the cliché... when one door closes another... In my case, being so much more homebound with David gives me more time to write.

"Promise you'll get more help," my daughter-in-law has been nagging me for a couple of years now.

I've resisted inviting — paying — a helper. Put off including a third person in our lives. My resolve is gradually eroding. For one glorious week Mary has come for an hour to feed David his breakfast. Stops me gagging on my food.

For the first time in years I spooned still warm boiled egg into my mouth without interruption.

Only a week to go before our dental holiday to Mexico, but this year for the first time I am hesitant, nervous of how the hell I'll cope. Don't want to accept David may be too disabled, and I cannot manage him alone anymore.

I see every swim potentially fatal, the journey a disaster and every meal out unmitigated hell. Better to cook in our room and dine on the balcony looking at the sunset. Nothing nicer. I'll take his walker for this trip. Borrow the hotel's wheelchair. But WHAT-IFS keep surfacing.

Idea. Change our one-bedroom to a two-bedroomed unit and invite a friend we both love and like. And that is what we've done. Just knowing she'll be with us means the pressure's off.

Here's to accepting help and that first margarita. *OLÉ.*

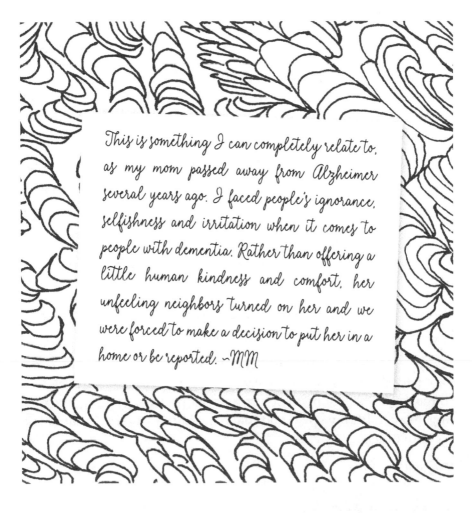

This is something I can completely relate to, as my mom passed away from Alzheimer several years ago. I faced people's ignorance, selfishness and irritation when it comes to people with dementia. Rather than offering a little human kindness and comfort, her unfeeling neighbors turned on her and we were forced to make a decision to put her in a home or be reported. ~MM

March 10, 2017

19. fly fly away

There are a hundred reasons why not to holiday abroad with David freezing and lurching as he does. An unwelcome stowaway, Parkinson's finds a way to show up wherever we travel. Guaranteed.

So he's not reported *INEBRIATED... UNFIT TO TRAVEL...* A constant fear of mine, I've slipped a yellow medi-alert bracelet around his wrist, and stuffed a card with his name and flight inside his shirt pocket.

I did lose him once. There one minute beside me at the gate, gone the next.

"He's wearing a navy cap with a large D emblazoned on the front," I explained wild eyed.

A security guy discovered him wandering, brought him back in the nick of time to board.

"Why do you do that to yourself? Are you nuts?" An acquaintance bugs me in an effort to put me off. It's not a question.

"What are a few hiccups and couple of hair-raising scrapes compared to the plusses—the pleasure we get from our travels?" I counter. "No telephone to bug me, no set routine, nothing like getting away to lift my spirit and make me human again. Great break for both of us."

Know it's true.

I think back to the month in Mexico: David and I lazing in a hammock strung high in the bamboo forest canopy swinging eye level with wild green and red parrots; our pre-dawn swims in velvet-black sea as the first rays of daylight skim the water's surface.

Least said the better about the inaccessible palapa accommodation we'd rented sight-unseen. Turned out it perched beside a disused Yelapa graveyard in the jungle... and that was just one holiday, one country.

My mind rambled to the Holy Man seated cross-legged beside the Ganges, the sacred ash he manifested for us to ingest.

Next moment I saw David and me in Chile soaking in volcanic water piped directly into a sunken pool in our bedroom... then us treading on strewn gladioli blossoms carpeting the steps to a Guatemalan chapel... then there we were floating on a lake one early sunset to watch flocks of Scarlet Ibis flying home to roost in Trinidad and... and...

"He's stuck in the lavatory." The BA flight steward roused me midway across the Atlantic. "Your husband needs your help,"

Hobson's choice in a case of either/or. Trapped. Poor David. Horribly humiliated, I found him with his pants around his ankles unable to hitch, zip and belt them up as well as being able to stand and open the door. Don't want that happening again.

Lesson learned: David wears elastic-waisted jogging pants while crisscrossing the skies. Wears an extra layer of protective underwear too.

"What about the actual travel, dealing with airports and such?" Nagging friend persists. "Surely that's too hard?"

"David rides to and from the gates in a wheelchair cutting lines like royalty. The assistant pusher just zips us through." Annoyed, defensive I didn't bother telling her that we have TSA pre-check, Global Entry and the like.

Makes me feel like royalty too. Pre-boarding getting to sit buckled in our seats before the scrum hits the aisle.

"I say if you can sit at home for hours staring at the TV, then why not in a plane? What's better than sitting tucked up in a reclining chair being attended to in the manner to which we wish, but were not born?" I snap at *Miss Kill-joy*.

I don't say its easy traveling with David disabled as he is, but neither of us are ready to be *stay-at-homes*. I'm grateful we can still pick up our bags and head out.

Yes, my duties as caregiver, and David's needs, remain the same... spooning food mouth-ward, counting pills, aiming and lifting limbs to arm and leg openings, moping urine spills etc., the grind of those twenty-four round the clock duties we Caregivers know only too well, will never, can never, change holiday, but using a trick or two we keep on rolling, rolling

I pull out my check-list.

1) Travel insurance: Yes. Don't forget this tip to add to your list, if you are planning a trip, Caregivers.

I discovered buying coverage at the same time as our tickets guaranteed acceptance–no questions asked. Confessing to pre-existing conditions, not required. But for that clause David might have waited months, a year even waiting to be cleared fit enough to fly home from France that year he was hospitalized for twenty days and so nearly died. Travel policy saved our butts. Paid a medical escort to deliver him to a New Mexico hospital bed.

2) Seat assignment 6a and 6d: Good.

Up front just behind Business Class. David should be able to walk that far safely on his own. And back out. Though once waiting to deplane, reaching into the overhead for his Carry-on bag, he teetered backwards taking down the line of passengers behind him like so many ninepins.

3) Wheelchair assistance: Yup, all arranged.

I have a wad of single, fives and tens stashed within easy access in a front pocket for handing out as tips. Often students, those wheelchair pusher guys are fun to talk to.

4) Pills counted and ready for fourteen days in their original pharmacy containers: Done.

I used to decant David's pills into smaller space saving containers. Big mistake. Seeing is believing apparently. Doctors just won't take my word for it. Seems they have to verify which formula of medication, what dosage, etc. for themselves.

*　　　*　　　*

I'm not one to fuss normally, but this upcoming trip to Puerto Vallarta has me nervous. Maybe I'm just old. Maybe the time has come for the vegetative slippers and fireside slumber. Perhaps I should have listened to the taxi man at Heathrow last summer. Been discouraged by the contracted thinking of that one friend.

I must give advice Mummy, let Daddy stay home. The elderly Indian taxi driver from Delhi at London's Heathrow shook his head watching me unclip David's seatbelt, and manhandle him from the cab.

"You're wrong," I replied, "It's kind of you to be so concerned but disabled as he is, my husband still gets pleasure from our travels."

"Misery-guts," I cursed, unsettled by the truth of his advice.

Projection? The start of our holiday was not a good beginning.

An adverse reaction to one of his medications, travel anxiety, not sure of the trigger, but something turned my normally gentle David paranoid.

Convinced I was trying to deny him his medication, he grabbed the phial of pills determined to take a double dose. Cajoling, fury, even threatening to call 911–nothing persuaded him to relax his grip.

It took two hours of what little night was left before I managed to trick him into giving them up. Sleep deprived and emotionally whacked out it was a miracle we made the pre-dawn flight.

David looked blank when I quizzed him next day. Had no inkling what I was talking about.

How different our lives. His. Mine. I liken him as a kite flying aloft and free, and me as the controller who yanks the string struggling to keep him earthbound.

Memories of the suicidally, *gawd-awful* night at the airport hotel, and the bruise ringing my wrist from his fingers, fading, the warm lassitude of being on holiday is finally creeping over me.

Sweaters and coats exchanged for shorts and shirts, and with sand between our toes, we flop recovering, massaged by the sound of the waves.

Question is, are two winter weeks at the beach worth the effort, worth the horrors it's taken to get to Mexico, I ponder.

Yes, so far, yes I say. Two weeks at the ocean does justify the means. Mind you, this might be IT–the very last time I travel with him alone.

Sleep deprived, and emotionally floundering, I came this close to packing David back into the car and driving home before we'd even started. Perhaps I should have listened to the taxi man at Heathrow.

Here on the beach in Puerto Vallarta, I watch him.

See David's face upturned to the sun; David drinking in the blaze of color as the red orb dips into the sea; David floating on his back lifted by the waves; David plunging into the sea.

Our skin tinged toast colored by the breeze off the sea, sitting on the sand together, David, our friend Jennifer from Colorado and me, a margarita in hand nibbling totopos and guacamole, As always in Mexico, Happy Hour is a happy hour indeed.

Each day a new day, I thank God for the gift of being alive.

March 18, 2017

20. reboot refresh

This holiday is a miracle worker. Haven't lost my temper for two whole weeks — worth the madcap scurry of journeying from snow-bound New Mexico to the beach heaven of Puerto Vallarta for simply that one benefit.

I'd forgotten how good it feels to be all sweetness and smiles, to coo instead of bark, to smooth my forehead un-furrowed. Will try to pack those feelings up and bring them home as souvenirs.

The nice calm person I used to be is creeping slowly back into my skin, the person who loves to idle and just BE. Gone the *hurry-hurry-we'll-be-late, get-your-shoes on nagger-me* at home who spins so fast I cannot breathe.

Back home, Cannot break free from the whirlwind schedule of hustling David to and from warm water exercise class, chair'robics, choir and…

"All your own doing," I hear you saying.

I can't disagree. *To slow down* has been my aim for years.

Ever since I heard my Guru's voice command me just that during meditation at least twenty-five long year's ago.

Slow down. Everything will come to you when you slow down.

I know I should, and I try, I really do, but intention and the doing of are two opposites I've not yet been able to meld.

Strange. I love the empty quiet I find when I am alone, when I wander the cholla cactus of the New Mexican desert, or perch still in some high isolated spot as I loved doing as a child, so why is it so hard to bring SLOW into what I call real life – i.e. my life as a house-holder and caregiver?

The answer, because I'm one plain, ordinary human, that's why.

From the balcony over breakfast, the sea beckons, but unlike other years I'm in no rush to gather my towel and dash down to the beach desperate to snag a deckchair before they're all gobbled up.

We'll find what we want, *no worries,* as the Aussies say. The sea won't dry up. The sand won't blow away. I smile to myself, content to calmly wait with my coffee and b-r-e-a-t-h-e till David comes to, and our friend emerges from her room.

Miss Sleeps-a-lot, I call her, envying her ability to conk right out at will, smile and relax, and wishing I could take not one page, but several, from her book. Hmm. A model I'll do my best to ape forever, I swear.

"How to box up this life and take it home?" I ask David. His eyes are closed.

I don't expect an answer. Don't get one, for he knows I know it's up to me.

I let him be.

I turn my face to the jungle-covered hills across the bay, watch palm-green fade to grey with the brightening of the day. Swim the slow pace of nothing.

We've visited the resort often enough to know which building, which floor, even which room has the best view and is furthest away from pool and restaurant noise. That way on David's OFF times when he's too on the wobble to make it to the beach, we can sit together on our balcony and contemplate, not a wall of other balconies, but the vastness of the ocean.

I count, "Five, six, seven, eight pelicans," watch them follow the swell of the waves beyond the swimmers.

A hut on an isolated beach no longer an option, a resort is not exactly quiet with its daily *rah-rah-happy-snappy* megaphoned happenings throughout the day, but for David with his Parkinson's, holidaying at one is a necessary trade off.

Wide paved areas make for trip-free, and walker, wheelchair friendly movement. The surroundings are familiar. David feels safe. What's more David is just another guest in need there. Fits right in. Can't say taking David on holiday leaves me worry free, but limitations of the resort aside, being dropped into this other world is pure heaven. I can even let down my watchdog role a little.

"Wait here," I'd command leaving him, mouth, often hung vacantly open, standing draped with beach towels while I located the perfect shade spot on the beach for us to spend the morning. Inevitably someone was standing with him by the time I returned

"I thought he must be lost," they'd say, kindly, though occasionally accusingly as if I'd abandoned him forever.

I'm talking of last year when we managed, just the two of us. This year, hurrah hurrah, I'll not be dealing with him for the two weeks entirely on my own — our friend is joining us. I lighten at the very thought.

Half dead from travel and the hellish night in Albuquerque, David stumbled from the taxicab. In a second the staff had him sitting in a wheelchair with a glass of water while I checked us in. Didn't even have to ask or for someone to help push him to our room.

"Keep the wheelchair for the duration of your stay. No charge."

Our friend not arriving until the next day, I'd been dreading dragging David downstairs to the outdoor restaurant, envisioning my struggle to seat him and get him up. Driving him in the wheelchair right to the table made the trip a doddle. I resolved to overcome my/our prejudice and get his wheelchair out of the shed when we returned home.

I thought back to last year to uneven pavements and sidewalks, to David pushing his walker, his dice with death, our race against the changing traffic lights to reach the supermarket across the road. How sometimes, I was forced to leave him on his own rather than trundle him across that speed track of a highway.

One afternoon, I deposited him at the entrance of the hotel with instructions to wait upstairs till I got back. Room key tucked into his pocket, I scurried off and food shopped for the best part of an hour.

Was he there when I returned? No, of course not.

The room empty, David was nowhere to be seen. Panic-dashing to our corridor on the forth floor I spotted a huddle of about half a dozen people slowly herding David with his walker and stopping at every door. Not remembering which room was his, the group was slowly wending its way from floor to floor trying his key in every lock. Felt bad of course. Guilt ridden for my stupidity in assuming he would retain the number of our room.

Last year was too hard. I swore not to take David on holiday alone again. I must be learning something, for this year we are three — the perfect combo for us. Forget, two's company, three's a crowd.

Yes, sharing space with a third person brings perspective to the way David and I are living our lives. How blinkered we've become to the subtle adaptations we've made under the silent weight of Parkinson's.

Me, a mutterer, talking into thin air I bounce words at David because waiting for his reply often takes too damn long. I've guessed the end of each slow annunciated word along the careful sentence, way before it's finished. Anyway, too often he gives no answer. Not easy to admit, but it's clear I've become a selfish loner set on doing, talking as and when I please, even riding roughshod over David's preferences.

Guess that makes me anti-social. Isolation can do that to a person I've read somewhere. I don't actually live alone at home, yet in many ways I do.

Having a companion, a normal person, our friend, *Miss Sleeps-a-lot*, with us, changes this year's vacation to two whole weeks of joy. I haven't laughed so much, talked so much for years.

I'd forgotten the fun of sharing simple tasks like prepping and cooking food, of asking another person how they would prefer something done — the novel experience of a two-way conversation, listening and giving space for the other to speak, the stimulation of receiving answer to a question, or an informed opinion on whatever subject we are chattering on about.

With my Boss-General's boots abandoned out of sight in the darkest regions of the cupboard, I am free to slop about as me. Be a regular foot soldier.

Thank you, dear friend, *Miss Sleeps-a-lot*, for sharing our holiday with us. Helping David and me loosen up and to pop back into our human skin.

And to think this holiday is partly free thanks to the cost-saving dental work we've done here in Mexico.

> I want you to know how profoundly your blog has affected me. I have chosen for the last few mornings to get up earlier and have my time clearing out the dishwasher, having a coffee and looking at the ocean, eating breakfast before I wake him up. . Once he is awake it is the endless run run run.. But you know what? This morning I was grateful that I could give him breakfast at the table and he ate everything because after reading your breakfast routine I realize how I should be thankful for these moments in the here and now. ~CC.

21. can this be happening?

Whether it was tiredness traveling back from Mexico that affected David, or just a Parkinson's muddle-brain, that caused him to double dose his pills yesterday, who knows, but double dose he did.

"Why David, why?" I yelled, aghast. "You never take two lots of pills at the same time. You know that."

But it was too late. He had. Gone and gobbled up his afternoon and evening pills together in one swift swoop.

Now I understood why he was *gone* keeled lopsided in his chair, eyes closed. Thankfully what he'd swallowed wasn't dangerous. Meant he'd stay semi comatose the rest of the afternoon and evening. Maddening.

As one small way of David having charge over his own life, I've left pill-taking up to him. Until now that is. I keep tabs of course, counting out and separating each dose into bright colored plastic lids saved from mayonnaise, peanut and other jars. Made it easy, or so I thought. Wrong.

Hate demeaning him this way, but from now on I'm taking over. Sideways watch him pop each pill. Hide the containers even. I cannot risk him doubling his seizure medication again.

"And just when he was doing so well," I muttered more disappointed than worried. "And now this, damn it. Hours of him being a complete goner."

Incapable as a drunk, at bedtime I had to help David stand, get to his room and undress, and lift his legs up onto the bed. Felt ill hooking out the partials from his mouth.

"Oh well," was my thinking, "he'll be fine in the morning after sleeping them off."

Not so lucky. One a.m. I heard him moving. Found him fully dressed, shoes on, wallet and keys in his pocket, flashlight in hand.

"Going somewhere? It's the middle of the night, darling. Get undressed and back to Bed."

"The man, the Leader... " David fumbled for a name, "... said to throw things in a bag and get the hell out."

It took ten, fifteen minutes smooth talking to get him to compromise and let me remove his shoes. Not his clothes though. Those he refused to let me touch.

"I am tired," I lied, "Need to sit down... thirsty, need water."

"Here," he said calming down and handing me a glass.

Then agreeing to lie down beside me, fully dressed he fell asleep gripping the flashlight tight to his chest.

"Sleep well? He asked next morning remembering nothing of the incident.

Nor did he recall interacting — more accurately, NOT interacting with the Immigration Officer.

At Dallas airport on our return journey, the Immigration officer alarmed by the grimaces playing on David's face, his lopsided, immobile slouch in the wheelchair, the man kept pushing me. He wanted different answers. Clearly I was covering up the real reason.

"What's the matter with him. Is he in pain? Why is he making such a face? Why are his eyes shut? Why isn't he sitting upright? Why isn't he speaking?"

"No. He's not in pain," I answered. "My husband's just tired from travel. He has Parkinson's and cannot control his facial expressions. It's a symptom called Parkinson's mask."

For one scary moment I feared he would deny David entry. I smiled attempting to calm him. Must have worked.

But note the red flag, people. Carry a Doctor's note certifying SAFE TO TRAVEL. I know I will next time we fly.

It was thanks in part to our friend *Miss Sleeps-a-lot* sharing space with us down in Mexico that the miracle began.

*   *   *

"I hope you don't mind me saying, but I've noticed a pattern," she ventured. "David conks out within half an hour of taking his pills."

Actually the pill — switch-off connection was something I had wondered about before but not fully taken in — the same phenomenon our son and daughter-in-law had remarked on over a year ago during a visit. I suppose I needed to hear the same thing more than once for it to sink in.

If you hear it twice — listen, goes a friend's dictum.

Nothing drastic, nothing dangerous, next day David put off taking his morning dose till his tremors started up and bothered him.

After all, I reasoned, David is still a doctor, even if the last time he'd worked was twenty plus years ago. He is qualified to make an informed choice. He knows his facial dyskinesia could increase. Joint stiffness, tremor and other symptoms too.

Trade-off is something only David can decide. Anyway, no way to know without trying.

Naturally I'm not talking monkeying about with life and death medications, those essential ones that must be taken religiously as prescribed. No. No. No. I'm talking of lessening the frequency and dosage of those tremor-controlling pills that were possibly knocking David flat.

I recorded the time: One o'clock, three hours later than prescribed.

True to pattern, half-an hour later he slumped sideways eyes shut. It took an hour before he was up and about and open-eyed enough to walk with us to the beach, swim beside us in the sea.

Anyone remember the film *Awakening*? Well David's *return* was something like that. Set me wondering: Had too many pills inadvertently been knocking him out?

I cringed thinking of the wasted hours. Wept for the time lost.

He. I. We. Intricately bound, be it in pain or joy, what one feels, so does the other.

I began a medication reaction journal that very morning noting milligram dosage, per diam-frequency, timing, and onset of any reaction.

Alert. Comatose. Eyes-open. Closed. Something concrete to show the specialist at his follow-up appointment next month.

Alert. Alert. I scrawled. My mind ran circles.

Can this be happening?

David's bouts of normal irrefutably increased? Wow — a positive effect of taking the new seizure medication? Could it be because we'd reduced his Parkinson's Dopamine medication? No matter the cause, for the moment we seized on the miracle was happening.

David-husband and best friend stared around with eyes so wide I could even see the color of them again.

"Hello there, my blue-eyed husband," I smiled. "Welcome back."

So it seems giving input to the specialists re Pill management is yet another way of being pro-active. After all it is I, his caregiver who is his day-in-day-out-eyes-and-ears. I, and all us caregivers, should at least be free to make minor medication changes don't you'd think?

Take warning though. Should anything go wrong, it's we who'll be blamed if things turned really bad. Accused of neglect even.

Watch out for state guardianship. The powers officials can invoke with a stroke of the pen.

I heard a scary story last week. A friend of a friend of a friend told of the one she loved, her partner of fifteen years, being snatched from her care — his bank account as well. Terrifying scenario.

One wrong word, one false report from one disgruntled relative and this could be David's and my fate.

I picked up the phone, okay-ed the medication changes with his neurologist.

I played the whispering game passing on the anecdote to the woman sitting next to me at our Parkinson's Action group. She'd complained of her husband's pill-zonked out connection. Same as David's. She was already juggling. Dosages. Timings.

"I'm just not giving him all the pills the doctors told me I should any more. All they do is make him sleep. He can't even speak." She complained. "I'm sure what he's taking is too much."

Was I stupid for not having the insight to experiment years ago? I suppose I took the importance of following the specialist's instructions literally. A lame excuse? Maybe. Never mind the past. We're on it now. AND the difference is amazing.

We had a real to and fro conversation yesterday. He carried the salad bowl outside for lunch outside, scanned the local paper and announced,

"I'd like to hear this Mahler concert, would you like to go?"

I was so startled, excited by his volunteering something without prompting, I bought tickets on the spot.

Hope. Ah, there's a teaser. I'm beginning to believe David can partly re-incarnate as he was before Parkinson's. Is it so foolish to want back the man I married? Chase after hope.

"Maybe with drug management... ?"

Every little glimpse of David as he used to be warms me. A few days ago days he talked so much, a friend stayed visiting for an extra thirty minutes for the shear pleasure of listening.

Today David put on his shoes and socks. Carried out the trash and helped unload the dishwasher.

This afternoon when he retreated unresponsive for two hours, I was forced to face reality.

His amazing comeback cannot, and never will be for all time and forever. Nor his dementia, physical limitations ever vanish. But each second he open his eyes, each second of lucid conversation is a second I can cherish.

Hope is back. Can this be happening I ask? Know it is. Yes, I see small miracles are happening.

Thank you C. It's really comforting to know I'm not out there alone, and that my blog resonated with you. I can picture you both overlooking the sea watching the tide recede and advance...sort of like our moods, and our husband's on/off times don't you think? A friend who was widowed over twenty years ago, once remarked, Better make the most of eachother while you can, as there'll likely be more years alone than you have left together." Hmm. That pulled me up short in mid moan. ~Liz

April 1, 2017

22. hate when...

The hell of this past week is nothing I want revisited on me again. You see, the man I love is sick.

Hate is a strong word. Inappropriate even. One I rarely use, but... well there always is a but isn't there... and mine is, I hate when David gets sick. The fuss he makes. Can't abide it.

Parkinson's symptoms I've gotten used to. Deal with them day in day out. But on top of that — David sick — not one more thing can I deal with. Moaning for example.

"Suffering is something to get on with alone," I was brought up to believe.

"No heed for that nonsense." At boarding school Nurse Moley, starched as the apron and headdress she sported, spoke harshly.

And I'd stifle any groan, clutch the hot water bottle that eased my monthly agony and bury my head in my pillow. That's British stiff upper lip for you.

Malingering will not to be tolerated, Nurse Moley's face read. Anything to break the monotony of the classroom, I remember rinsing my mouth with hot water hoping to fool the thermometer and claim a sick note.

But, back to David. Oh dear. I sound as harsh as Nurse Moley ever did. I shame-facedly admit I am — at least on the outside. Inside I hurt. Struggled for breath as he struggled. I don't quite know how to disguise the rising terror, this was IT, his final illness, and he would slide from me to the next world.

I'm just not hard-wired with a gentle hand. Wish I were like Florence Nightingale though, and gifted with her touch. Supposedly, to be a good parent a child needs modeling. Ditto to be a good nurse.

It began five days ago. First a lowering of his voice by an octave after Choir, then a cough, followed by him emitting loud moans as if he were about to expire.

"David," I snapped. "No point sitting here. Why don't you go to bed if you feel that bad. It's just a chesty flu'."

Wrapped in a green wool shawl knitted by his mother more than thirty years ago, David looked so sorry for himself. I fetched a heat pad. Laid it on his chest. Fed him ibuprofen even though his brow was cool to the touch. Poured lemonade and made him drink. Checked he was in no pain.

"Keep warm and sweat it out." I order, when really I want to comfort with, "I'm sorry you are sick, my darling."

It was if a lump grew where my heart should be. I fled to the living room turned up the volume of the TV. Hated myself for the stone stopping my mouth from speaking kind words.

A confusing mix: anger, concern, desperation, fear, deep anxiety, spun into one inseparable swill.

I quashed the image of a parent-less girl, sick, isolated in an attic room of the Children's Home, the 8th birthday she spent whispering to her cloth dog. Kissing his nose. I still hurt for her, seek the comfort she sought. Tap the hard shell with which she covered herself. Covered me.

Next day after David fell ill, Monday, I called for a doctor's appointment. Fat chance of scoring.

"I'll try to get him in next Thursday," the receptionist cooed. I put down the phone. Said not a word. Too nicely brought up to sneer.

"Thanks for nothing. That's three whole miserable days ahead. What if he developed pneumonia? He could be gone by then."

Should I, shouldn't I take him to Urgent Care? In the meantime should I, shouldn't I give him those four leftover antibiotics I unearthed from the freezer?

"You know better than that," I admonished myself. Couldn't bring myself to throw them out though, so put them back. "Just in case."

I watched him carefully. Took his temperature, fed him soup. Thursday came.

"That's it. Get up. We're off to Urgent Care."

David never stirred. No way could I get him to sit up. Much less trundle him to the car.

Only one thing to do — call 911.

"What service do you require? Is he breathing?"

Describing him — his closed eyes, impassive face, the stillness of his body unleashed a flood of tears. Contrary to our conversations about readiness and letting go and the DNR documents we'd both signed, at the moment I voiced his symptoms I knew unequivocally I was not yet ready to let him go.

Not uttering a sound, he squeezed the EMT's finger. Showed us he was still there.

At the ER David's eyes opened after 5-plus hours of IV fluids and Oxygen. Can't say he was as right as rain but right enough to come home.

How fragile life is. How unexpected death. For all my talk, I realize I'll never be prepared.

I tell you these details to show the emotional currents I, as a caregiver, ride. Para-gliders, suspended high in the air never knowing where an invisible down draft will suddenly slam me.

Minor as this incident may be, it felled me helpless. Home, David slept like a babe. I fitfully.

As if he'd never been ill, next morning, David was up, dressed himself, pulled on his own shoes and socks. He cleared the breakfast table...

Given one more day together, we spent it quietly. Sat a little in the spring sunshine.

"I thought you really were exiting this time," I ventured.

"No. My visa was denied." Coyly, David smiled.

*   *   *

Friday, the sound of a whistle filtered my dreams. Staggering from bed, I discovered David on the tiled floor jammed between the bath and bedroom.

"I've been here nearly an hour. I'm not hurt but I can't get up."

It took a mighty effort; me pushing, sliding him on the bathmat; David scooting, till finally he could reach up, grasp the basin and heave to his feet.

"Why didn't you call me sooner the minute you fell?" I scolded, hating to think of him uncomfortable and cold. Nurse Moley again — speaking through me.

"I didn't want to wake you," he said.

Was I hearing right?

The weekend passed. Monday, alert and rearing to go, I readied him for swim class. Fool that I am, I held his swim bag in one hand, took David's hand with my other. Began walking the flagstone path to the gate. Somehow he missed his footing and crashed face down off the path onto the gravel.

Shocked, David lay planted, stuck, his temple half an inch from the razor sharp corner of a granite rock. Too spread-eagled and awkwardly angled no way could I move him. No way could he.

The neighbor and I managed in the end. Slid a yoga belt under his arms and yanked.

Two falls in as many days. Then David's ER drama. I am whacked out. Emotionally and physically numb. See what I meant about para-gliding?

What did I miss? How much was my fault? Why didn't I lead him by both hands, use the walker, use the wheelchair? Did I give him his pills too soon, too late? Am I asking too much of him pushing him to all these classes? Why do I react to his sickness so negatively? Why do I turn into a sergeant major?

The post mortem began. Could continue forever. Telling myself, be kind to yourself, no one's perfect, just doesn't cut it.

David is fine, walking, talking, watching TV, back to himself.

Me? My back aches. I'm catching his cough and feel like SHIT.

Yes, a caregiver's life… that's what I've got.

Liz, my loneliness feels different now that I have read your blog. I thought I was going mad, was selfish, was unkind, was feeling so tired and having no time to do anything other than take care of the man I love. Your words are so relative to my existence. They give me comfort. ~CC

April, 8, 2017

23. what if...?

After sitting with David in the ER last week I got thinking. What if I was the one carted off to hospital unconscious? What would happen to David? Would the EMT's take him along in the ambulance and have him admitted too? They surely wouldn't just leave someone so clearly disabled to fend for himself home-alone.

Worry. Worry. My mind raced. Hadn't thought of this WHAT IF before. But I'm now spurred into getting some practical plan in order about his care.

I imagined the worst scenario: David slumped sideways, his eyes frozen closed, unable to phone for help. No food. No water. Perhaps lying on the floor for days. Not so farfetched as one would suppose.

Only three years ago a friend in the village felled by a stroke, lay semi-paralyzed and helpless for thirty-six long hours before a worried friend called the cops and he was discovered. I was across the road from his house that night at a yoga class in the Community Center. Felt such guilt being so near and yet unaware of his distress.

I lay awake. Wracked by a bout of coughing. Damn. My turn. Must have caught whatever dreadful chest thing David suffered last week.

What if this morphed into pneumonia… then what? The list of *what ifs* multiplied in my head leaving little room for sleep.

I woke to the crippling symptoms of flu.

In its fog our young Ayurvedic doctor's wise words floated to me from seven years ago, when David and I spent a month in a Kerala Ayruvedic Nursing Home.

Rest. Be quiet. If a disease appears, allow it to do its work then move along. I remembered her smile. Her politeness. Her way of saying,

Don't fight. Lie still and allow the sickness to pass. You Westerners... she chided, *The minute it turns hot you rush for an iced drink, switch on the A/C... but a dog? What does he do? He lies in the shade. Keeps very still.*

Easy to say but no such chance with David to tend to. Of course I should have stayed in bed tucked up warm to sleep and sweat it off. Instead forcing to my feet I moaned,

"Done it before. Can do it again."

Could it be fifty years ago?

I saw myself a single Mum and three months pregnant, my face swollen with mumps dragging out of bed to care for my toddler firstborn with no family in sight, and my then-husband sailing the China seas and far away. And I, a Navy wife newly posted to Australia not knowing anybody yet.

But here in New Mexico I do have friends. In hindsight I could have/should have phoned around, but... well, at the time it seemed so feeble.

Truth is, the thought of asking someone to please take David off my hands never entered my head. That damn British hang-up again I suppose. Just can't shake it. Help for David? Yes. I'm only too happy to accept. But help me? My toes curl at the thought. Yet... how I'd have welcomed a gift of steaming chicken soup.

I had a roll-over accident once. Hung upside down, held by my safety belt. Now why couldn't I simply say, "Help me please. Just get me out of here and quick?" Instead of...

"I'm stuck," I hesitantly told the stranger's face peering through the car window. "Do you think you could help me? I don't seem to be able to release my belt?"

"Of course," the stranger said amazed, crawling inside through the window releasing me.

Back to last week's boring flu. Day two, reluctantly I rose from my bed, off-loaded David at his Acupuncture appointment and swim class. Was I daft that I didn't cancel? What made his needs more important than mine?

Turned up the car heater and slept curled in the front seat counting the seconds till I could be home and lie flat. The wind howled from the East threatening snow. Finally home, I helped David battle from the car and propelled him along the path. No relief yet. The daily routine clamored.

"You need to rest," David said, "to get your fever down." His hand lay gently on my shoulder. "What's for lunch?"

"And how... may I ask?" I snorted under my breath looking round for the invisible helper who could take over. "Who do you think will... "

David meant kindly. No point arguing. Zipped my mouth. Snatched catnaps when I could.

Better now, I once again tussle my what if scenarios. Scribble down my what I want to know is... questions.

"What Emergency protocol is in place for David's safe care if I'm not there?" I asked our Doctor's receptionist. "Pretend the worst and I'm unable to communicate."

"Good question," she paused. "He would not be allowed to ride the ambulance... hmm. And he needs 24 hour care? Problem."

I asked the guy from Senior Services.

"Tricky question," he pondered. "There's nothing. You have to make your own arrangements." He shrugged his shoulders.

I asked the caregivers at the Parkinson's Coalition. "Compile a list. Tack it behind the front door. Or pack a VIAL OF LIFE with information and store it in the refrigerator."

The local fire department agreed to have someone stay with David till the contact person arrived.

Contact person... Top Priority... Passwords... unravel... I penciled placing the slip of paper in the growing MUST-DO pile. Will... check. Power of attorney... set up. Respite Care... arrange...

"STOP. Just listen to yourself," my inner voice roared. "Do what you need to do, then drop it."

That was it. In mid worry I stopped. Can't believe how negative I had become — a worrier, even. How far off my center I'd wandered.

I looked over. At peace, David sat still in his chair. No wonder the leader of our Grand Canyon river raft trip awarded him the Buddha prize. Mine? The most improved camper. And that was fifteen years ago at least. Skirting whirlpools of icy water, un-fazed, David clung to the dinghy's rope, rode the rapids, and lazed when we were becalmed.

When we landed ashore each evening, David and a like-minded guide settled crossed-legged on the sand puffing smoke clouds towards the raging river, while the rest of the party, me included, scrambled the rocks on wild hikes, hunted waterfalls, gathered sticks and...

Hmm, I could be like that dog the Ayurvedic doctor spoke of. Or follow my David's example.

I inhaled a long, slow breath.

April, 15, 2017

24. hanuman and i have a birthday

I lost my power, you might have noticed from last week's blog. Sickness. David's, mine.

Sucked into an ugly mire of heat pads, diapers, cold cures and tissues, I lost sight of UNCONDITIONAL LOVE. My physical strength gone, floundering in a whiteout of exhaustion and rage, caregiving loomed black.

The thought of dental plates floating in a glass, me having to fish for, and help David fit them turned my stomach. Swabbing smashed glasses and very sticky drinks two nights running, when all I wanted was to curl up under my blankie with a glass of hot lemon and honey, and be miserable, became insufferably impossible.

I mean who cares about such little accidents and chores? Not me normally.

"That's another glass gone, another spill. One yesterday, one today. How many times do I have to remind you?... PUT THE DAMN GLASS DOWN between sips." With that said, I burst into tears.

This was no way to live... me shouting, David miserable. How could I have allowed such a nasty me-person into my skin? I resolved to about face and scramble back into my body before I forgot where I kept my inner peace. What happened to the four gates of speech I used to practice?

My words nowadays were neither *kind, true, nor necessary.*

While David still slept, sitting before my puja — my altar —set beneath my bedroom window, I lit a candle. The flame wavered in the cold stream of air preceding the dawn. A new day. But one I vowed, would like the sky, fill with light.

Change the prescription of your glasses, fingering the rose tinted spectacles I kept as a reminder, my meditation teacher's, my Guru's words returned. But how? To actually see differently — David, our lives, my caregiving — not so easy.

I recalled my month-long Ashram stays in the 80s and 90s, the sweetness of silence and meditative calm, the lake I'd walk by, the saint-statued gardens I strolled. I was nicer then, could be now again if my householder's life outside its womb-like walls were as carefree I grumbled. What I'd give to recapture a little of its feel, the person wandering there…

I pictured David as he used to be. Imagined how I would feel, if like him, I lost my independence. I thought of his temperament, how placid and accepting; the relentless symptoms of Parkinson's disease, the dark cloud he moves in, the blueness of his eyes when they popped open.

He must be a saint to put up with so much, with me, my quirks, yet still love and thank me.

I noticed my mood shift as I listed the happy moments that kept us going. Yes, we were lucky comparatively speaking. Positives definitely out numbered negatives.

Caregiving didn't seem so bad. It was me and my attitude I must change. What was the quote? The one saying there's no point moving your deckchair around on the Titanic? Got it.

In two days I'd turn 79. On each birthday I like to think-walk my life. "Thank you for my birth," I always begin. "Thank you, David," is how I end. "Thank you for being my husband."

Today would have been my father's hundred and seventh birthday if he'd lived. I rarely saw him ruffled or heard his voice rage.

Had he always been easy going like that? Not growing up together,

I saw an eccentric romantic — a man to idolize.

"Get dressed quickly," I remember him calling me once when my brother and I were visiting him in Devonshire. I was maybe nine or ten. "The sun's shining," and off across the heather moors we scurried after him.

Coming across a stream, in a flash his clothes were off and he was rolling in its icy water.

"Come on in, the water's glorious," he called.

He was right. It was. Did the same with my children, "Come on you Pussy feet," I once yelled, "Follow me." And I dipped in and out without a stitch. Brrr, this was New Year's Day on the Devonshire coast of freezing England. The sea, the sand beneath my feet so cold I lost all feeling in my legs.

My father developed a liking for watercress — in just one afternoon, he dug a pond, re-routed a stream, constructed a waterfall to tumble oxygen into its water, pushed the plants' roots deep into its mud impatient for them to mature enough to fill a sandwich. An Aries, impulsive, his nature attractively childlike, ideas never stayed ideas for long. I'm like him in many ways, but placid I am not.

David awoke. Called for my help. I blew out the candle, stubbed out the incense stick and stood.

"Think calm," I willed myself.

Holding the mantra in my mind, I popped David into the shower and helped him dress. Decided I should give myself some time off.

David's sitter arrived, not for a couple of hours but for one complete and glorious day. It was Hanuman's Jayanti, his birthday celebration. A monkey-God's birthday? I guess he, like me, could celebrate one. Hanuman, the Perfect Servant, the perfect servant I strove to be, but never could. The Perfect Servant, for him I named my blog.

Years back one summer in the Ashram I became curious... Did the Guru sleep in an iron cot, on a feather down bed? Was the bedroom luxurious, like a cell or... In a dream Hanuman appeared, sat up in a golden space where the Guru would have lain, briefly pulled back the sheets before lying back and covering the bed. Protector of privacy, protector of his mistress, loyal and perfect servant — Hanuman — oh, to be like him.

Two hours drive and I drew up to the Hanuman Temple in Taos founded by Ram Dass of the book "BE HERE NOW."

Ram Dass was in his eighties when I heard him speak in Santa Fe eleven years ago. Struggling with word-finding after his stroke the word hospice worker eluded his tongue. "Err... err... A DEATH MIDWIFE," he triumphantly declared. Could there be a phrase more apt?

Waiting for Ram's program to begin, a persistent unseen voice insisted I buy a raffle ticket for a flight to India.

"You will win," the voice said, "and you will go to India."

So convinced was I, I bought not a book of tickets, but a single ticket. Who won? Yes, me. I was the winner. I laughed with gratitude.

A month later David and I flew up and away to Kerala. Unbelievable luck? A lesson in listening? I choose the latter.

Once in the Temple's grounds, I dropped back into India.

Swept into the culture of my birth in a swirl of silk and gold-edged saris. I wormed through the East Indian crowd surrounding the temple. Not an inch of space in the sea of bodies inside. A man leaving pushed past me as I peered through the door. Delicately picking my way like a crane I pounced for his vacated square foot of space.

A Harmonium in front of me, a drum either side, bells and cymbals clanging, the crowd's ecstatic chants, all thoughts were hammered from my head. David, me, my weariness — blasted.

Nothing existed but the roars of devotion. Nothing existed beyond those sacred walls but the song of emptiness. And in its emptiness I slipped back into my skin.

The final two hours of the twenty-four hour-long chanting closed with the deep calls of conch shells, jangling bells and cheers.

Eyes shining like those around me, connected in love, I stepped into the sunshine.

The gift of another year ahead, I have new resolutions make and to keep.

Serve as Hanuman Served, read the quote displayed on the wall.

Everything you describe reinforces my conviction we caregivers are normal humans pushed into doing what does not come naturally. I love that you travel as we do, brave the vagaries of non-handicapped hotels and restaurants. Hurrah, we're alive, and making the best of our shitty situation. Take care of yourself" they all say. Sends me mad as it does you.~ Liz.

25. Happy and Glorious

David-as-he-used-to-be returned on Easter Sunday. His eyes opened wide and his mind sparked alert. A new beginning? Dare I believe? Was it premature to give thanks? Just having him back for even a single day was miracle enough to have me singing. Him too I imagine. Whether the quirk of a GOOD day or the result of the new reduced medication regime, I'd take it, whatever the reason.

"Look David," I said at breakfast pointing to his place, "A rabbit."

And I smiled watching his surprise, then as he ripped the foil and bit off the bunny's chocolate ears.

The phone rang, and via Skype, my grandson in France held up a day-old fluffy bundle of a cheeping yellow chick in his hands.

"Happy Easter, Granny," the five year old sang "It pecked its way out of its egg this morning."

From the kitchen window I wondered at the confetti of pink blossoms that escaped the hard freeze, the pair of bluebirds frantic nest-building in the bird house tacked to the fencepost. And I feel again the same childish excitement I felt on finding a stork had flown through the window the night before Easter and laid the most beautiful chocolate egg inside my topi — Indian helmet — I'd placed at the foot of my bed.

In Devon, as a child fresh from India, I remember the feel of the first skinny-legged lamb I'd ever held, the softness of its woolen curls, the pinkness of its tongue, its pathetic bleating.

Every spring the fields along the high-hedged lanes mushroomed white with ewes and their lambs, and wriggling tails as the newborns knelt to suckle, then skitter off and really skip, really frolic. I'd hang over the gate clapping at their antics and wishing I could play with them. Here, in the New Mexico desert, I miss that.

An April baby, born in spring, *Let this year be full of joy,* I pray each Easter, and fill every vase in the house with yellow daffodils.

When I was still a newcomer to the States the girlfriend coming to lunch today, and I joined the pilgrimage to the Sanctuario in Chimayo Wanting to arrive at the church on Easter Sunday we set off at dawn. Still dark, at four in the morning silent penitents limped beside us, blistered, weary from their all night march.

On the final mile where the road twists through the cactus spotted hills, rounding a bend remember I stopped in my tracks—saw the sun rising on my right, and the full moon hanging low in the brightening sky to my left. I spread my arms wide — the moon balanced in one hand, the sun in my other. Each Easter, I return to that moment, the joy bursting.

Back to yesterday's wonderful UP day. David's resurrection.

Shaved, dressed a clean poppy-red T-shirt, he was hovering, waiting for our friends to arrive.

"Would you like to help?" I asked.

David unwrapped the Cotswold and Brie cheeses and set them on the board.

"Anything else?" He asked, counting out four forks, four knives to lay the table.

"Happy belated birthday. Happy Easter."

With armfuls of tulips and daffodils, our friends burst through the door and into the garden. Sparkling wine, Shishito peppers and potato chips beneath the leafing peach tree, this was the life.

My mood relaxed, became euphoric even.

No spills. No smashed glass. Spring green leafing shade. First hummingbird darting. Skin warming. I was in heaven. And Parkinson's was just an ugly dream. I threw an olive pit far into the desert. Listened to David chatting favorite jazz musicians with Mr. Musicman, as I call my friend's husband.

"I'm just checking," David said pointing. "… if you see elephants stomping there beyond the fence?"

"No we can't see them. Are they still there?" They inquired without a twitch of an eyebrow.

It's difficult for the non-disabled and their caregivers to understand the joy of such an afternoon… of being normal… of a meal where messy eating is ignored… of genuine friendship… of good company and laughter.

But until the age of eleven when loving guardians took my brother and me in, there were no times spent like this — a meal — Mother, Father, brother, me around one table. At least this is the story I've told myself.

EGG

On the shelf above the boy's bed sits an egg.

A chocolate Easter egg a full eight inches high. Mottled, dull, its surface proclaims its age.

For three years the girl, his older sister, eyed that egg.

Sometimes when the boy wasn't around, she licked her finger and careful not to leave a furrow, ran it wet around the base stealing just a little taste.

The shelf above her bed was empty save for a scantily clad bronze woman statue on bended knee holding an orb of frosted glass.

The girl's egg was smashed and gobbled the same day it arrived, its contents of sugar almonds quickly hidden in a secret place. If she didn't eat them, someone else would like the urchins in the compound where she and her brother lived guarded by a witch when she was nearly six, her brother three.

"Do you have any money?" The urchins had asked. "We know the secret to make coins grow. Double." They'd grinned. "You must bury and water them for a week."

And she had.

The two of them, dispossessed of all they knew, all they owned, eventually sailed for their Motherland, a land they had never known where at Easter the children gathered yellow gorse petals from the moor, and onion-skins from the compost bucket beneath the kitchen table, to tightly wrap in squares of rag around white-shelled eggs laid by hens and color them.

Chocolate eggs were unknown in the place, a paying orphanage, where their father left them while he re-turned abroad to earn a living.

The boy chewed his collars and wet his bed. The girl wet too, had nightmares, and like a cat turned feral.

Then a miracle occurred. A family took the boy and girl and tucked them warm beneath soft eiderdowns in a room where just the two of them slept, and gave them each a toothbrush of their own. Pink. Blue. Face cloths were no longer shared. The boy no longer sucked his collars. The girl, tamed, no longer screamed.

The first Easter with the family, the boy and girl woke to find a stork had flown through the open window and laid two chocolate eggs in the nests they'd built at the foot of their beds just as storks had done, they remembered, in India.

Ribbons, gold lace-paper, silver coins, icing flowers, a yellow sugar chick. The boy placed his egg on the shelf above his bed. Guarded the precious thing that was his alone. The girl, now wiser, gobbled every speck.

*   *   *

The guests gone. Early evening. We were alone.

I looked up. David was singing.

By the light of the silvery moon we'll hug and spoon…

I can relate so much to the "always being on guard, one ear to the ground, one foot ready to leap up" syndrome. Our friends and acquaintances are much more aware of this than we think and luckily they allow for it. Doesn't take much to bring a tear to my eye on a given day —depende del dia! ~Carol

April, 29. 2017

26. high time

"You need to get away. really away. Have some time to your self,"
my friendly advisor, the doctor's receptionist peered over her specs
handing over the renewal application form for my Handicapped
Driver's Pass.

I must have made a face, for she added, "You won't like what I'm
going to tell you, but I mean not for a night but for one whole week.
Check David into respite care and… you don't have to go away, stay
at home and get your house back to the way it used to be. The way
you like it."

I pictured the disarray, the coffee stains on the pale green living
room upholstery, and the fringes of our rugs kicked ragged, the
extra unsightly trash bin in the bathroom, the closet bulging with
protective underwear.

Sorry, caregivers, I still can't bring myself to use the word *diaper.*
Too demeaning. Too brutal in connection with my husband. All
adults for that matter. It's a hang-up I tussle with.

The Receptionist had a point. Our *feng-shui* home had slid horribly
un-feng-shui. I shivered.

My father would have dies if he were alive… Chairs askew off-cen-
tered. Pictures on the tilt. Squished toothpaste worms hardening
in the basin. Socks tossed smelly littering the floor. Dishes piled
lopsided on the counter.

"You can judge a person by the order of their home," he declared. "Crooked pictures and stopped clocks particularly"

I heard his voice every time something out of place caught my eye as I shuffled David by, too weary to care about some neat-nick ideal at the expense of David's comfort and safety. I mean really, what the hell does a little crooked matter?

Yes, the life I now lived revolved around David... his calls for help, his needs, his timetable. Mine? No idea. Dropped someplace I've long forgotten.

Too often, just as I am settling into meditation, or still blissfully asleep, am in mid attack deleting unwanted spam, have my hands full of wet laundry, am half way to the trash bin, or sitting at the computer expanding some thought to add to my blog, I hear...

"I'm stuck. I need help."

Or my brain alarms David's medication was overdue, we were late for swim class, his acupuncture appointment...

No matter. David's and my first night apart was fast approaching. One whole night, a motel on the sunny border of New Mexico down south, a banquet, cruising uninterrupted for 400 miles, I could hardly wait for an evening and a whole night to myself away from it all.

Then it came. The time to part. Fussing like a mother seeing her child off on a school bus for the first time, I pre – and re – counted pills, laid out David's clothes, wrote instructions for his sitter to cover every unlikely calamity. Even how to lift and swing his legs to get him into bed. How ridiculous was that?

FUSS. FUSS. FUSS. KISS. KISS and...

One more and another farewell kiss.

Suddenly David looked frail, pathetic even, so vulnerable. How could I be so awful as to leave him and pry the two of us apart, glued together as we were, like moistened postage stamps? The sitter wouldn't know how David liked his breakfast fruit cut, how many spoons of yoghurt to add, his little fads and fancies...

"David likes the curtains pulled at night... " I lingered, thoughts running.

What if he died and I wasn't with him? If I had a crash? If... He must have read my mind.

"Oh, for goodness sake stop. You'll have a wonderful time. Go enjoy yourself. I'll be fine. Just go. GO ON GO." David hugged me, kissed my lips, gave me a little shove.

"Bye, darling. Bye. See you tomorrow... "

I jumped into my girl friend's car careful not to glance back. *Out of sight out of mind* they say. And it was.

Turn-taking the wheel every two hours, munching the tomato sandwich I'd made, the cube of cheddar cheese, as we drove along, and chattering non-stop through the towns of Socorro, Truth or Consequences, Hatch, it seemed but a minute before we veered away from Las Cruces off I-25's speedway and into Billy-the-Kid's village of Mesilla.

The motel was perfect. I had only my own suitcase to carry and unpack, only myself to shower, and primp ready for a night on the town. Well hardly that... hardly wild. My friend and I arriving too early at the venue, too early for a salt rimmed glass of Margarita, too early for the Awards Banquet where Sam Donaldson, the TV celebrity, would be the key-note speaker, we circled the Historic Plaza killing time.

For a moment I thought how it might have been with David, of all the difficulties dealing with his disabilities. He might have tripped on the pavement, closed his eyes against the setting sun, frozen im-mobile, never made the steps leading up into the church. I checked myself.

I was here with a friend. No worries. No stress. I looked around. The long evening shadows, the shafts of sunlight between the cot-tonwoods patterning the Square, the Victorian wrought-iron band-stand, the setting, couldn't have charmed me more.

A stretch limo pulled alongside the pavement spilling a group of a dozen High Schoolers; young men smart in coal-black shirts and pants sporting startling Mexican-yellow suspenders, a Graduation Queen in bridal white and her yellow tu-tued Maids of Honor for a photo session in the bandstand. Outshone, I watched two elderly musicians pick up the tin can and blanket at their feet, his guitar, her tambourine.

I wondered for how many evenings the old couple sat together on that same bench performing for coins, the joy of music. Their youth gone, the red silk flower in her hair now faded, her girlish curls now grey and straggly, the grubby white lace of her dress hung too young for her wizened frame, she walked slowly, stiff beside her husband. Stooped beneath a traditional wide Mexican gold braided hat, he too walked bent.

I watched them limp away, sweethearts still. I like to think they loved each other, saw still the beauty that first attracted them to wed.

I wished my David by my side. Wished he sat here on the bench with me. Wished years of togetherness together.

We have agreed that if and when the time comes, we won't allow the medicos to make decisions for us. Your defiance is inspiring.
Thank you, DdV

May 6, 2017

27. change?... as good as a rest?

Or so goes the adage. I was looking forward to these 8 days in Arizona cheating the bitter winds of New Mexico... a rented condo, no landline, the two of us in summer cotton and shorts soaking up a little warm between visits to the Movement Disorder Clinic.

"Might as well squeeze in some fun even if you are wired into your E.E.G. hat," I enthused to David knowing eight days of doctor's tests and therapists' visits would hardly be jolly.

I felt just a smidgen of guilt for having taken off to the Mesilla banquet the week before without him.

With good timing, now right on its heels, here we were, the two of us off to Arizona and some warmth.

Warmth we got. 101°F today. 103°F predicted for tomorrow. 105°F the day after.

"Remember that egg, David? The time we fried it on the rock in a butter pat from the motel?"

"Well we tried," David giggled recalling how it sizzled nicely, then slithered into the dust before we could eat it.

I attacked Google Maps and planned day trips... see the cacti in bloom, explore the Tonto National Forest, watch kids tubing in the Salt River, swim the Saguaro Lake, discover Frank Lloyd Wright's innovative housing, and marvel at one of the tallest fountains in the world shoot 360 feet into the air on the hour. Oh yes, I had our free time between doc visits all planned.

We knew the routine from the first time four months back — what he could, and could not do burdened by terminals stuck to his scalp, trailing wires, a battery pack on his back and me following him with a camera. More of a nuisance than a hindrance but we knew he'd at least be mobile.

The temperature soared to 108°F throwing my plans to hell. No matter. David was the reason we were here — tests, evaluations, and consultations to better his life. NO MORE SEIZURES David's brain read-out showed, thanks to the new meds.

Just to discover that wonderful result made the effort worthwhile; the long car drive, the hours of google-search for a condo, the packing, the strain of bundling David in and out of restrooms along the way, the chivvying to get him to his appointments on time.

The neurologist clapped his hands unable to contain his delight at the lively exchange he and David were sharing.

"Now you are so incredibly more alert I think you'd be a good candidate for… " and he explained the benefits of some new injectable medication. Didn't sound too attractive to David, even less to me, his caregiver. Needles and I are not compatible.

"It's a rescue remedy for his off times," he enthused. "At least hear what the initiating nurse has to say and take the free trial dose while David's reaction can be monitored."

I said WE. Ooops, slip of the tongue. Caught myself too late. Not so off actually.

Yup, caregivers suffer their partner's disease. Differently I grant. I may not have Parkinson's, but Parkinson's governs every damn second of my life. Yup. That's the truth of it. David's condition makes him tremor. The tremors I suffer are from rage. His face is mask-like. I have to wear a mask to hide what I feel. I could go on. And on. Another day perhaps but back to Phoenix.

"Usually I give you a nice package, a CD, leaflets and stuff." The nurse opened a bag displaying vials and needles.

We stared in horror as the nurse screwed one to the other and stuck a cushion with a needle.

"Now your turn," she said. "Pinch and cinch." At least I think that's what she cooed.

I eyed David's shaky hands, his struggle to drop in the vial and set the dial to the correct dose. Let's face it this was a task he could never do. OK. I see it's his caregiver's job. MINE damn blast it. But I never signed up for this.

"Give me that." I took the paraphernalia from him. "I can see I'm the one who will have to do the deed," I sighed blanching.

Stabbing a cushion was one thing. Pinching and sticking David's belly flesh with the real medication made me squirm. Emotionally I mean. Was this something I as his wife could ever take on? David? Did he want such an invasive procedure as part of his life?

The magic potion knocked him insensible. No way could he be roused till the drug wore off an hour later. NOT the reaction the doctor or nurse expected. Not the magic tremor-free awakening we'd fantasized.

That night at four am I startled awake with the streetlight jiggling though the blinds of the rented condo. The mattress was moving, shaking. But it wasn't an earthquake it was David. His tremoring. His mind working overtime.

"Are you awake? Are you worrying about today, darling?" I whispered. Funny how one whispers in the dark. "What are you thinking?"

We turned towards one another. Compared to that injected medication to control tremors, pill-taking didn't seem so bad. But it wasn't me taking them.

"You have so much more ON times these last four months since taking the seizure medication, why compromise what's working. So what if you fall asleep after taking a whole pill. We'll cut the damn thing in half and see how that works. If you could live with that then I can."

He took and swallowed a whole *carbo/leva dopa* pill, stopped shaking and slept like a baby till breakfast.

Then it was up and another dash to the clinic. I must have been crazy to have imagined this trip would be a holiday; the heat, the stark landscape rigid with saguaro giants demarking the suburban highways, the weed-free meridians, the prison-like walls around sterile properties. Mind you we both loved the tropical air at night, the exotic flame trees and bougainvillea.

We did manage one whole day off. Appointment free. David's daughter flew in from Washington State to visit to her dad. After helping me peel off the hat she drove us through the barren land to Saguaro Lake. I wanted a picnic. I wanted a swim. A real swim. The condo pool didn't count. A few boats stationary with fishermen rocked far offshore. Not a person in the water.

I stood ankle deep in the lake on the stone beach a little distance from an old man heron. Waited until he spread his massive grey wings, and lifted slowly into the air before I waded in and rolled ecstatic in the water's cool.

A brush fire closed the road to my planned picnic spot. Just as well, for the sun burned fiercely by then, enough to melt the hardboiled eggs, heat the Rose wine, and wilt the salad. Thank goodness for A/C and indoor picnics for that is where we, and our stuffed cooler ended up.

May 13, 2017

28. it's a long way to...

It's not the destination, it's the getting there that is the thing.

I used to love driving the American highways. One hand on the wheel, music gently ironing flat the blacktop to an oily sheen, while composing plans that will never make it past the dreaming.

Today's drive will continue till day's end. I am conscious of my breath coming slow and steady as the speed set on cruise control. Lifting my accelerator foot off the pedal, I flex my instep and stamp-tap the floor. A bare ninety miles lie behind me.

Keeping my eye on the road, I ease my neck with a head roll, and scan the rise where the road dives out of sight between the cut. Guess fifteen miles to reach it. Check the odometer. Wrong. Smile. I'm two and a half miles short. I roll down the window sniff the blast of delicious hot, then roll it quickly shut again and flip the a/c vent onto my face. Red cliffs tell me I'm near the Indian Scout, Kit Carson's cave. Plan on taking a detour to see it my very next trip.

I'm cruising I-40, Route 66, through the Dine, the Navajo land towards Gallup. Imagine the ugly smell of the ill-famed lock-up for drunks, and swerve away speeding onto the town's by-pass. Another hour yawns. Chalks up seventy miles.

SKY CITY, reads the sign. *ACOMA.* And I remember an early date with David — a Feast Day in August, a celebration so foreign to me then, new as I was from England: the contrast of the women's stiff wooden tablitas against the volcanic flow of their hair, the painted bodies of the men, the chink-clink of the dancers' silver bells, the beat of their moccasins stomping the bare ground, the vibration of the drumming... I still have the beaded memento David gave me, recall how happy the giving and receiving made us as he tied the leather thong about my neck. Swear to unearth it from my jewelry basket and wear it more often when we reach home.

I can't ask him if he remembers the tamales — "the best ever," he declared — bought from a food stall in a shady back ally, for David is sleeping.

Two hours ON, two hours OFF driving turn and turn about. That was how things used to be. Before Parkinson's snatched away his car keys. When shared driving — shared anything — was a possibility.

1984 was the year our lives collided on a dusty village Rodeo Ground in New Mexico — a Green-card carrying Canadian, a Green-card carrying Brit born in India, neither yet an American Citizen. A Child Psychiatrist, a sculptor, both twice married and divorced. Who could have imagined such a match?

David was super boss-leader then, the sole driver of his car, and my guide into the spangled milky skyway in which I'd been dropped from England's green and tidy hedgerows.

Oh those days of love... They're the memories that keep me going when I can see no further than the next duty I must perform. The next pill I must dole him, the next trip to the toilet I must help with, the appointment to drive him to, and...

That was then. This is now. Our roles flipped, it's me who wears the boss-leader's hat today.

Can't imagine the me I was then, the timid mouse who needed to learn to become American and voice both her wants and don't-wants, and the years it took before our roles settled equal. Different colors, same styles, but otherwise our hats perfectly matching.

His. Hers. If I could snatch the constraining cover from my head, I'd throw the damnable thing as far as the wind could take it.

I can't. I am David's lifeline to the world he opened for me but now cannot reach unaided.

The drive from Phoenix to our village in New Mexico looms a long eight hours my mind fussing how we'd cope just the two of us alone. The pre-dawn air at 4 a.m. was already hotting up. Condo to car, condo to car, our bags, groceries, the unwieldy walker, and cold-box, snacks and bottled water, weigh heavy in my sleepy state. I haul the bag of trash to the dumpster, haul David last. Got him safely down the ramp. Eyes closed, pulling back, he stands frozen beside the passenger door.

"Come On. Come On. MOVE. GET IN damn it. We're wasting time." Desperation grips me by the throat.

The lockbox for the condo key is too stiff for me to open. Not even a dog-walker about to help. I give up, place the key on the kitchen counter, pull to the unlocked door and flee. It's almost six.

"We're an hour late," I fume at my new best friend, Siri, the GPS lady. "Turn north onto Fountain Hills Drive. In three miles make a left onto Shea towards the Beeline Highway. 499 miles remaining to your destination." GPS lady soothes.

A beginning. An end. A finite distance.

Phoenix to home. I'll be there by four. But caregiving? My role as Caregiver? I stare at the unfolding blacktop stretching to the rise ahead. See no end. Surmounting the crest the road twists and dives into a steep curve. I brake to begin my descent. The gear grinds. Gives a lurch. The grass-covered caldera on the valley floor is green and wide. Then up the other side I climb again. The saguaro cactus sentinels wait for us on the crest. Mute. Watch as we pass.

I reach what promises to be the final rise, I see another horizon calling, yet still no destination.

David's head is back. Face dreamy, he sleeps. I am driving alone.

May 20, 2017

29. Missing Something...

I must be missing something about the charms of Caregiving. *CHARMS?*

Perhaps I am blinkered or just plain incompetent, for that is how the old friend I was chatting to on the phone made me feel. Mind you we'd not been in touch for a year at least, for she lives abroad now, so perhaps had only an inkling of how our lives were running. I looked to excuse her, and be halfway forgiving.

"Oh, I found caregiving so rewarding," she cooed. "I don't regret a single moment of that wonderful time I gave to mother," she paused allowing silence.

Was that a dig at me? An implication of my failing? Did she want me to tell her how wonderful she was? Wonderful? Not the adjective I'd use. What planet did she hail from?

"Yes, caring for mother was such a gift," she added, or some similarly smug comment.

Was this some kind of competition? If so I wasn't playing. Just couldn't bring myself to counter with my truth.

I pictured her: Red Riding Hood doling sweetness from her goody basket... taking her mother on shopping trips or for drives in the bluebell woods, cooking meals and performing other gentle daughterly duties.

"You must have made your Mum happy," I replied feeling increasingly inadequate with every word. "But she could speak couldn't she?" I returned a little sourly. "... still able to carry a conversation... dine out with friends... feed and walk unaided... and was continent... use the phone... and could... ?"

If she picked up the underlying bitterness in what I was saying, she didn't let on. Had the woman ANY idea what David and I were dealing with?

"Well, lady friend... ever experience any caregiving moments like ours this morning?" Never voiced any such bitchy comment of course, and let her rattle on.

Well, you can tell I'm grouchy as hell today. Somehow bludgeoned by my friend's lofty attitude. It's not as though David and I don't have wonderful moments, for we do, but caregiving wonderful, and some new-age mumbo-jumbo gift?

Let's have a reality check here. Bloody hard work is what caregiving is. 24 hour duty. 365 days a year. I mean really — so rewarding — indeed. You mean clothing, wet and soiled; food, spilled and smashed; limbs, bruised and cut; David, upset and helpless: me wrung out of smiles and... ?

The muscles of my upper arms and shoulders throbbed, my lower back twinged when I moved. So far the day had not gone well. I wasn't in the best of moods to listen to a load of codswallop. But let me backtrack and maybe you'll understand why.

It was six thirty a.m. when I heard David's whistle. Its call didn't sound urgent.

"I'm dressing. Be with you in a minute," I responded unhurried, pondering if it was warm enough to wear a cotton skirt, and if my yellow blouse would be a good match. "Give me ten seconds."

I found him crouched naked, his body toppled half under the bedside table and between the bed. The mat beneath him sodden.

"God Almighty," I bellowed covering my fright and running to him. "Oh, darling, how ever long have you been here?"

"Three-quarters of an hour… " his voice came faint. Exhausted.

"What! Why, oh why the hell didn't you call?" I cried in anguish. "Let's think. Let's think this through. How to get you up? Meanwhile at least let's get you warm… " and I managed to pull a T-shirt over his head, thread his arms through the sleeves. "Gosh, they're so heavy, David. Can you help please and P-U-S-H."

As much as I tried positioning his limbs so he could kneel dog-gie-style and then heave up against the bed, he couldn't budge.

"Bend this leg," I tapped his knee. "Flatten this foot. Come on. Now MOVE." But despite all my effort, all my guidance, his knees remained folded, locked, his legs stiff and as unwieldy as an oar out of its rollock. David stayed stuck.

"Relax. Relax, can you? Stop fighting. I'm trying to help." He wasn't resisting of course. The rigidity of his muscles just felt like it.

Defeated, I lay panting on his bed.

"I'll have to phone our tenant." The phone rang and rang. No help there.

"OK. Let's give it one more go before calling the EMTs. They'll get you up and make you comfortable."

David refused.

It took another half-hour to get David halfway onto bed. He lay face down not speaking, legs jutting into the air, and arms folded useless beneath his chest. If I left him like that he might easily slither back to the floor, I worried.

"What to do? What to do?" I spoke aloud searching for inspiration. "Ah." And I yanked the edge of the blanket beneath him and rolled him flat onto his back.

Half an hour later David stood upright on his feet and walked into the kitchen unaided. That's Parkinson's for you, one minute he's OFF, the next ON.

It was breakfast time. We drank our coffee wrapped in silence mulling over the two golden rules we'd violated: David had got out of bed without anyone being with him: I had struggled and hurt myself when I should have waited for help.

So many falls: first the flowerbed three weeks back, now this second one; then there were the three or four evenings when he forgot how to get up from his chair, and couldn't remember what limb he needed to move to get into bed; and those occasions when my physical strength and verbal instructions weren't quite enough to jumpstart him... we were in crisis.

Neither of us willing to face the truth that going it alone was sometimes and more frequently impossible, we spent the day barely speaking.

Was it time to call in Hospice care? Would they give us more help? Should we look for a full-time helper? What to do to be more safe while preserving his autonomy? All day questions battled unspoken. Should have installed a Baby Monitor, should have woken, should... should... Didn't help me feel any less defeated and inadequate.

Mid afternoon the phone rang.

"Thought I'd give you a buzz," the girlfriend I hadn't spoken to for a year hailed cheerfully from the old country.

How-are-you-I'm-well-thanks exchanges and other social niceties over, she launched onto the joys of caregiving.

I walked to the bedroom and lay flat on my bed, moved the receiver away from my ear, laid it on my chest microphone up, and closed my eyes. My friend was still talking, complaining.

I hadn't the nerve to say, "you had it good." And, "If David had all the faculties your mother had — was a walking, talking living doll, so to speak — " I too might see the rewarding charms of caregiving."

"Who do you see of the old crowd?" Innocently meant, her question brought to mind our dining table set with two places. David's. Mine.

"No-one, really. Socializing is too hard nowadays. For us. For them. But for a few really close friends, we keep to ourselves mostly... Sorry I'll have to go. I see the guy from Senior Services coming up the drive," I lied to cut her OFF.

Neither of us good at expressing our feelings out loud I spent the rest of the day darting to and fro from den to the living room to check on him. David stared ahead, his eyes on the TV. Unseeing, it looked to me. I guessed his thoughts were tumbling like mine.

I rubbed his swollen foot and ankle with castor oil positioning it beneath an ice-pack on the walker placed in front of his chair.

"For the edema," I soothed. "How does that feel?"

My way to show I still loved him. He held both my hands. Squeezed them. His way of showing.

David's snoring and muttering noises called me to his room.

Hoping for some profound wisdom or significant words from the sleeping oracles, instead he began to laugh and laugh. I stood by his bedside, the light from the corridor outside his room playing on his sleeping form. Serene and peaceful as a child's, his face was creased with a smile so broad the corners of his mouth lifted opening his mouth like a crescent quarter orange — an expression I hadn't seen David make for perhaps fifteen years thanks to his Parkinson's mask.

I caught the pleasure of his mood and overcome with happiness I began to smile and laugh. Then his voice broke to a trembled cry. Still asleep he rose to sitting and reached towards some unseen person.

"Lie down, darling. You're sleeping," I whispered tenderly.

Stroking his forehead he calmed.

May 27, 2017

30. are we there yet?

We called Hospice the day after our crisis, after David fell, and my struggles to get him up so nearly failed and did me in, the day when barely a word passed between us, and I'd spent it despondent and alone.

By alone I don't mean actually alone, I mean the alone-ness of doing for the man I love who's food stays on his plate untouched unless I fork it to his mouth, who's eyes cannot acknowledge my existence because they are sealed closed, who depressed, curls up inside himself. Silent.

"You don't have to be actually dying to call hospice for help," the doctor's receptionist explained when I asked her for names of the providers in our area.

"Interview several agencies and make sure they offer Home Health Care as well," she advised. "Just know Doctor will give his support if you did decide to go with hospice."

For two years David and I had pigeon-holed and marked the hospice option, "To be opened later."

Step one. We chose an agency at random, took the plunge and phoned.

"We're not sure if my husband's ready... we'd like some information... your criteria for taking someone on." I hesitated. "It may well be too soon."

The agency's Social Worker was free and would come round that afternoon.

"Just to talk, explain hospice services," she reassured.

Two hours of interview later, a folder of information under my arm, we watched her car disappear down the drive.

She'd failed to disguise her horror on finding David with his eyes frozen closed. Me, walking backwards, pulling on his hands and guiding him across the room to his chair. I could see she thought his need for Hospice Care a given, and David a fall-risk who should be in a wheelchair full time.

For the first hour she was with us David sat inert, his right leg spasmodically tremoring, eyes shut, nodding his head, occasionally murmuring to show he was alive.

"Damn," I castigated myself. "I shouldn't have given him his Parkinson's meds so close on her visit." On reflection it was good the Social Worker saw him when he switched off.

"Have you thought about a commode beside his bed… using boards to slide him from bed to a wheelchair? He should wear the yoga belt at least, and you… " Her sentence hung unfinished her eyes wide.

C-O-N-F-U-S-I-N-G.

David transfigured into a sentient human. Fully back, eyes popped open, and with a clear voice he asked an informed question.

"Would Hospice require me to stop receiving care from my neurologist?" David paused.

"Swimming? Choir group? His ping-pong?" I added. "Chair aerobics at the Senior Center? Walks to the mailbox? The Parkinson's Think Big And Loud Physiotherapy? Would he be allowed to leave the house for those?"

Without actually telling us *verboten*, the Social Worker hedged. It became clear, to qualify for their program they expected David to be virtually housebound.

We thanked her for her time, smiled, shook hands and saw her to her car.

David and I looked at one another.

"Well?" I asked. "I'm not there yet," David sounded cheerful.

"Hurrah. That's my opinion too. Gosh, I'm so relieved." I said slipping my arm through his.

It was as if one hundred redwing blackbirds flew in celebration round our heads.

Just the realization David wasn't yet ready for hospice reignited our hope. We still had a life to live, "and miles to go before we sleep" — to plagiarize the poet, Robert Frost.

We weren't there yet and *choice* was still an option...

... to walk alone, with or without a walker, a wheelchair or use hiking poles; to sleep in a regular bed, sit in a regular chair, use a regular toilet, roam the house and creep off to his den at will. Then there was our traveling... I listed all the good things going in David's life, the many things David can, and still plans to do. Fly to France this summer and spend time with the family for one thing.

I don't mean to imply David is fit, able and together, for each day, each hour of the day, each minute, for without warning and just when I'm gratefully thinking he is so normal, so able, Parkinson's might flip him helplessly disabled. Him onto his metaphorical back, and me, into an emotional vortex. I still can't get it — the not knowing.

I felt like cheering as the social worker turned onto the main road, and could have leapt over our rooftop, I felt so light. He was alive and wanted to live.

"What about going up the road for lunch. I don't feel like cooking," I said and kissed the top of David's head — easy to do now his six-foot has shrunk curves towards his feet.

Energized, David slid out of the car by himself and walked to the café table unaided, picked up the menu and ordered Caesar salad and a Reuben sandwich.

"How about a glass of wine?" He suggested.

Was I sitting opposite the same sad creature I'd found curled on the floor the previous day?

Something changed. We smiled more. Brushed fingers. Saw hope in each other's eyes. Watched less rubbish on the box. Sat outside in our favorite shade spot beneath the peach tree, laughed at the single fruit clinging to our one-peach tree.

Suddenly the days weren't long enough.

"Let's plan on doing more together. What about going to the Highland Games at the Balloon Park this weekend?" I queried.

Grabbing sun hats, water, and David's walker we spent the day steeped in Celtic music — Scottish, Irish and Welsh. The keel of the bagpipes, the thrump of boron and drum, the strains of, "... *By yon bonnie lass and by yon bonnie brae... the bonnie, bonnie banks of Loch Lomond,*" gripped us ecstatic. Perched on a narrow picnic bench we tasted *Haggis,* and watched men stagger trying to balance the caber before tossing it end over end.

Among the band of marchers, I watched a kilted woman steer her motorized wheelchair one handed and pump the Bagpipes under her armpit with the other, her cheeks puffed red from making music.

"Wow, David, look at her go. Isn't she something," I said pointing her out.

She stretched a swollen leg to the ground and scooted her foot to better position herself. If she was in pain she ignored it. That woman was doing what she loved and having fun.

Oh, for David and I to have her determination and spend more time doing what we enjoyed. Nothing fancy, spend a whole afternoon reading, or listening to a CD, perhaps see a film, take a couple of drives, eat an ice-cream on the Plaza, or go to more events like this.

Back home a couple of days later, tired, I inadvertently clicked an icon on my computer and brought up something called Live Chat.

Gave myself one horrid shock. There in front of me I saw myself as others must... a wrinkled, tight-lipped, harried woman... Nobody I'd want to be around. God, I looked a fright.

"If you make a face like that it will stick."

So it was true what adults scolded at the Children's Home. From the look of my scowling face, it had. Stuck. Better unstick it fast, and smile, was my thought.

That evening on the T.V. I heard an expert describe an unexpected side effect of Botox.... *people with depression felt happier, less depressed after being injected in the forehead...* the man went on to explain. A botox-smoothed brow tricked the psyche into believing it was un-worried: no-frown-therefore-I must-be-happy philosophy.

I'd better get smiling. Maybe by smoothing away my scowl with a make-a-happy-face-and-feel-happy philosophy, and holding myself proudly, I would trick my mood. I straightened my back elongating my spine and neck, and strained to lift the corners of my mouth, glancing in the car's mirror to check.

Did I imagine it, or did I feel less tense?

Some days I think, I can't do this any more, so many years lay ahead with no improvement possible. I am lonely even though I am not alone and your piece sometimes helps me and in a way empowers me. I thank you for that.. ~Jt

June 3, 2017

31. to voice or not to voice...
i'm talking feelings here

I have no idea what, if anything, you and David feel about his Parkinson's. A friend's harsh judgment stunned me.

Do you share your feelings — ever? She continued. *I never hear you mention them. I don't see how your marriage has any intimacy if you don't share,* she pushed me for an answer.

Wordless, I stared digesting her words.

Not even a fly on our wall, and she dares rank the intimacy of our relationship. Not any of her business anyway. Maybe unnatural to her, un-American even, but David, a psychiatrist, and me a Brit, holding back works for us — a successful ruse that keeps us from drowning beneath the weight of the *PAR-KIN-SON'S* stones we carry with us day and night.

I mean who wants all that American express-your-feelings stuff anyway? Not me. Nor David either.

Worn down — too plain tired for more than flop after a chore-filled day, what this caregiver craves is a soft cushioned armchair, my feet up, and my mind stopped with television's blanket, and possibly a glass of Pinot Noir.

The last thing I want to deal with is emotional spillage.

Mine. David's.

"Each to their own," I murmured, defensively to my friend.

"A buttoned lip works for us."

I've long given up asking David the meaning of my night's dream like I did way back when we first shacked up and thought he, a psychiatrist, would find it riveting.

"It's too much like my work," David stopped me in mid whatever fantasy I was relating. "I don't want to hear it."

I'm glad he did. Oh, the yawning boredom of listening to another's ramble dribbling on about the symbolism of this and that image. I admit I'm intolerant.

Today I am working on the Eastern dictum:

Speech should pass through four gates:

IS IT TRUE?
IS IT KIND?
IS IT NECESSARY?
IS THIS THE RIGHT TIME?

Saves David and I a lot of grief. Another saying that fits our lives — the way we communicate: *One look can speak a thousand words.*

Yes, those ancient philosophers knew a thing or two, as people in love can attest. Anger, gratitude, sadness, guilt, shame take but a glance. Comfort takes but a wordless cuddle. And David gives great cuddles.

My friend's criticism got me thinking. Stirred up thoughts I keep mostly private. All that chitter-chat she calls intimacy, the-let-it-all-hang out variety, would send me stark staring nuts if I was forced to be around it.

"One time I stayed overnight with a couple of friends," I related to my friend. "In mid-anecdote the wife happened to lift an eyebrow while her husband was talking. *What do you mean by that?* He rounded pouncing. Her *nothing* denial, failing to satisfy him, set him dissecting each imagined nuance insisting *tell me, tell me, I can see you're feeling something.* She was being attentive that's all. Finally she lost it and exploded into tears with rage. Poor woman living with a man who couldn't shut up."

All that talk-talking invading my calm. Hate it. Love David's quiet. Love silence. The beauty he shows me.

"We, David and I, have an unspoken pact," I tried to explain. "It suits us not to splatter our private misery and fear into the others lap–so why open your mouth?"

But sharing is intimate. My friend stood her ground.

David and I are both sharply aware of the inevitable, the Parkinson's slurry slithering slowly to annihilate us. Knowing is terrible enough without voicing it. Blubbering the day long about the million little upsets only creates more hurt to my mind.

Least said soonest mended may be a cliché but it works for me. I can't bear either of us rattling on about minor upsets and hurt feelings when one look at our faces, or a gesture says it all.

Most times talking to David is like talking to the man in the moon. Head back, eyes closed he shows no reaction when I tell him THINGS I want to share, or dangle the new shirt I bought for him before his chair. I could take offence. Cry hurt. Instead I have to make do with knowing he's heard and he may want to see it the next day.

Some nights my mind runs havoc blocking sleep and I feel he and I are prisoners trapped in an iron cage waiting to drown in the incoming tide. Hardly helpful for David to hear such a horrible thought, or of the messed visions I have of his future and inevitable creeping end. Selfish, cruel even, to DUMP my garbage into his ear and make him feel a failure as my husband, my companion.

If all I can say is, "God, isn't this Parkinson's just awful?" thoughts — feelings, if you insist — are much better kept to myself.

Caregiver-me's job is to give him a reason to live.

"We've had a lovely day," I encourage as we head for bed.

"We have enough good times to make life worthwhile, don't we, David?" I ask seeking reassurance his believes life is still worth living.

"Many," his lips move.

I feel, yes I *feel*, so good when he affirms he's okay.

I love our silent telepathic intimacy that knows what the other feels without *mouth-speak.* Fills me with happy.

I'm thinking of the New Mexican nights David shook me awake with a "get up, get up, get your slippers, come just as you are," and I'd stumble naked to snuggle beside him under a duvet in silence to count each star as it shot free from the Milky Way. Then trace the shadows to the village down the hill to the moonlight spotlighting the church spire.

No need for words to share our feelings.

I remind him sometimes. "Remember... ?" I ask, thumbing an album, how happy you look. David stares from the page, a coconut in one hand, machete raised, exchanging smiles through the camera's lens. His cheeks glow pink as the hibiscus flower behind his ear.

I feel your pain, frustration, disappointment and each time I read your blog I realize that will be me in the future. Every single minute of the day we are aware of our situation, there is not one moment that I feel free, me, happy, without responsibility. How did this happen to our loved ones, how did it happen to me? ~CC

June 10, 2017

32. metamorphosis
... Grub to...?

Giving up? Giving in?

By comparing my first blogs to my more recent, it's clear I've morphed. The angry caregiver of then has mellowed, and my tongue now silver-coated compared to then. It's not that I'm a different person. Turned saintly or anything. Or become a better caregiver. I'm more resigned to my role, that's all.

"I'm my husband's full-time caregiver," is how I introduce myself now, though my lips don't always part in a smile as I say it.

Like poor Kafka's grub waking up one day with his bug persona struggling to be understood, I yearn for people to see and treat me as they did before.

How can they? I've become a Kafka-grub, all vestiges of wife-me, carefree-, independent-me, artist, regular, ordinary-me, gone, completely gone.

"But I am still here," I try to cry out. "Look. Beneath this grub's skin, it's me just as ever I was before."

But unlike Kafka's grub who expired from hunger and melted into a slime never to recover, I have not remained helpless lying on my back waving and moaning uselessly as the creature. I'm steadily limping back one foot at a time.

Like it or not, babe, my thought runs, *a caregiver is who you are now.*

Better accept what is.

And as I do, oh so slowly, I feel myself giving in and my mood shifting back to almost normal — even great again. Really.

It seems by giving up the struggle to escape my caregiver's hell, a surprising calm is claiming back our home. I feel wisps of happiness returning — a happiness, which, like sun behind a cloud, has been merely hidden.

Did I disappear once a caregiver's hat was thrust on me? Turn me into a grub forever? And if not, who, or what am I? I'm puzzling that conundrum.

Giving up? Giving in? A subtle difference between the two perhaps, but I've discovered both are lifelines to my caregiver survival.

Surrender sounds so defeatist. Brings to mind my angry, "I can't do this any more," and, "I give up" cussing.

Some kinds of giving up are good, I've concluded. Sort of like New Year Resolutions,

I swear to give up railing and straining, and outbursts of, "Move Godammit," and "Lord give me patience."

I swear to never football his socks across the room again ever... my resolutions read like a list of shameful sins.

Makes me feel like a heel, and I hate when he says, "I'm sorry." For whatever he's apologizing is not his fault, not mine but the fault of his nightmare, unstoppable disease.

Poor David. How can he bear me? Bear living? You'd think I'd have got it by now, and given up begging him to do things he cannot. Like finding the car's door handle and dismounting double quick so I can drive into the garage. How handicapped he must feel to have me goad him on when his body won't move. That, I've already given up.

Preparing cold slaw for lunch one day last week, mortified by an earlier uncharacteristic — medication induced, I suspected — outburst of his, David stood silent by the kitchen table.

Watching. Contrite.

"Do you want anything?" I asked.

"Morphine," he answered softly. "But we don't have any, do we."

I dropped my knife and put my hand on his arm. "Oh David darling, why?"

"I'm ready for the long sleep." He stared not at me, but at his feet.

Coming out of the blue, his words were shocked hard to hear. I'm not ready to face David is tiring, weary-worn from enduring daily indignities in order to buy a little normalcy in his life. The burden of his dependence on me, and others, for the simplest of tasks such as heaving his dead weight into bed, pushing pills between his lips and, yes it's those dreaded teeth again, pulling them from his mouth. The toll those tasks take on us both.

We talked. I comforted him, for that is all there is to do. All either of us can. His mood lifted, and there's been no mention since of giving UP. And anyway why shouldn't David feel miserably hopeless sometimes? It's only natural after all. I know I would.

I dropped sad because he was, but gladdened we were able to discuss such a difficult subject.

I find some expectations easy to give up — the plain stupid kind like finding a birthday card propped at my place, or expecting David to call the plumber, fix the loose door hinge, pay the electric bill, change a light bulb, open a can of beans and perform other clichéd husbandly duties.

I still make plans though know they're liable to be broken. No point expecting them to unfurl smoothly.

Take Saturday for instance. The monthly meeting when David's caregiver takes over from me so I can take off before David wakes.

At the time when daylight had not yet revealed the cedar and piñon bushes pockmarking the land, I rose earlier than normal hoping to grab an hour of quietude before I left. The air hung delicious, and the rose bush outside the kitchen shimmered tangled strings of dew-pearls.

I stood in the open doorway hands cradling my coffee. Barely taken two sips, when David called wanting me to help him up.

No use grumbling. I turned back indoors. Gave in without a growl. Yup. Surrendered, if you will.

But don't interrupt me in mid boiled egg. Or fried, for that matter. To eat one whole egg uninterrupted is an expectation I cannot surrender. There is something about the delicate balance of egg-white to yolk, and the slow savoring every spoonful start to finish, on my own.

I don't quite know what childhood memory I dip into, but from the flipping over the hour-glass timer and setting the sand running, I'm into my ritual: blue and white egg-cup, matched saucer, silver egg-spoon at the ready, toast slathered with butter, from the first crack of the shell till the last lick of yolk.

No talking. No phone calls, No helping David with his food should he happen to appear. No jumping up for coffee.

… So nearly there, when David drops his knife and with it my *cloud-cuckoo* hope.

Wanting? Want this. Want that. Crazy-making. Demand ones rights? Win the Lottery? Right out of luck on that one. And wishing for David to again stand straight and tall, for our children to live close by, the world to spin in peace, and, and…

And the grass to be orange — you want that too? I ask myself.

A dream life is not what I've got. Nor David. Choice, I conclude is a luxury.

More and more often, I'm feeling like Mrs. Bee with her Dr. B, as she calls him, who rather than battle the outside world, hole up in their private beehive world safe, and happy. Truth is, David and I are finding we're less stressed when no eyes are upon us.

My David's an easy man to love. His sweet nature. His never ranting. His iron endurance rarely breaks down despite challenge after challenge. I wish I were as placid and had his take-things-in-your-stride philosophy. Instead, my mind knots frantic schemes to overcome one hardship and demeaning situation after another to make his life more tolerable.

Should I get out his watercolors and him painting again... put him on extended release caffeine pills to overcome his sleepiness... only cook with coconut oil... use more turmeric?

Foolish of me to dream David will one day be able to Frisbee Parkinson's away forever just because he is now so much more alert.

It's the start of a new semester at our Community College. It's back to our old routine — twice-weekly warm water swim class, twice-weekly physio, and lunching occasionally at the Senior Center and TV and a glass of wine of an evening.

One late afternoon last week we went for a stroll. David with his hiking poles, me swatting bugs with my hat. Together we slow-walked 0.4 of a mile through the village outskirts. His breath came hard and his body began trembling.

"I need to stop," he said accepting his energy limitation and giving in to his body's message.

David stayed where he was while I fetched the car. Instead of push-pushing till he collapsed, he listened to his body.

It was a lesson for me. One I'd do well learning, and in a hurry. Stress kills, they say, and too often stress is in my life.

Giving up in the negative sense, I haven't. GIVING IN in the positive sense, I have.

Mrs. Bee, wife, caregiver, whoever, right now, life ain't 'arf bad.

June 17, 2017

33. roller coaster

Breaking open one of two fortune cookies lying on the restaurant bill, I pulled the exposed slip of paper from the crumbled shell.

Although it feels like a roller coaster now, life will calm down.

"Yeah. Yeah. Right," my thoughts ran. "But when I'd like to know? And make it be soon, please, oh Fortune-cookie God."

I reached across the table for David's wrist, and turned his watch face towards me.

"Oops, we must be out of here in two minutes to make your one-thirty pedicure appointment. We'll have to pick up your prescriptions on the way home after a stop to mail your letter."

Wednesdays are full on. A six-thirty rise allows time enough to get David washed, dressed, and breakfasted before bundling him out of the house and into the car for the forty-minute drive to swim class. Gives us twenty minutes to bash ourselves awake over a game or two of ping-pong until his helper arrives. Takes his helper half-an hour get David undressed, showered, don swim trunks, and dip in the Jacuzzi for a quick warm-up before class. I'm usually starving by the time the two of them saunter into view clean and spruced freeing David and me to head for lunch.

Better than making a special trip to town, one time-and-motion cram-packed day is way preferable to me than wasting two.

Do double, accomplish double, in double time, is the mantra I work by.

Time being the currency here, the faster and the more I multi-task, the more time I earn to spend on the doing of absolutely nothing.

Okay, there are exceptions I have to confess, like when I balanced six jars of freshly canned jams onto the pile of laundry.

"Might as well save a trip."

Intent on dropping them off in the garage en route to the clothesline, I tripped, and… well, I don't need to describe the Jackson Pollack mess of glass, strawberry and white sheets. Yup, I should have re-membered it was the tortoise not the hare who won the race. And yes, I know the odious slogan more haste… that ends with less…

Perhaps a leftover from the idle-hands-make-mischief philosophy drummed into me as a child, even now if I snatch a feet-up-on-the-couch moment before the evening's five pm. clock-off time, I keep half an eye open ready to spring to my feet should someone peer round the door and catch me sinning,

I wish it wasn't so, but spare time nags like an empty shelf calls for a vase, a stack of books, or one of my sculptures to fill it, though what I really want is the empty purity of a minimalist. One of my life's quandaries considering my dreams of Zen-emptiness and yearning for utter quiet.

When I first moved into this house, below my living room window I created a half-moon expanse of white sand, empty but for three black basalt rocks and the patterns I raked. All remained pristine for the five months before the March winds blew. Scattered my con-templative calm to the mountains of the Pecos Wilderness.

I tell you this to show in my heart I'm Zen. Dreams cost nothing and I still cling to the intention of reaching its state one day.

Circumstance is what I have to thank for the madness in which I'm now caught. Nevertheless, all my life, from the igloo house I wove with twigs of willow and planted as a child, to the meditation cushion in my bedroom, I've built in periods and places of respite to counterbalance the frenetic rush of motherhood and my job.

Holding the six weeks of summer vacation before me as a carrot, I'd work my Speech Therapy job ten straight months, take unpaid leave, close-up the clinic, and walk away. Oh, the relief as our house door banged shut, and we left London's traffic headed for the channel and Spain—a mountain village tucked into the folds of the Picos de Europa. Camping gear, two adults, two children, seeing us emerge from our mini was as wondrous as a conjuring trick.

This is going back a bit. I'm talking the 70s and 80s, the eleven years we summered in heaven. No shops, no electricity or running water, no road beyond the lane leading to the village, no cars, no horses, not even a donkey, we slowed to the pace of the plodding cows, and the stork perched statue still on the church steeple.

We set camp in the meadow adjacent to the sprawl of red-roofed houses clustered around the "Lower Bar," one of two segregating the village — "Top Bar" for Franco's Catholics, versus the anti-establishment families down our end. Our Palacio de Algodon, Palace of Cotton, nestled in the tall grass half sheltered by the shade of four crab apple trees.

From our tent, the meadow before me stretched her furrowed strips of vegetables a clear quarter mile to the base of the Almonga's mountain scrub oak and granite.

The field, empty now in the evening, I watched the village women in their black, and the widower, Juanito with his hoe, pass through the rough oak gate and head for home, their baskets heavy with potatoes, onions, bunches of carrots, and perhaps a frilled leafed cabbage head.

The ragout of lamb simmered in a blackened pot above the fire's embers. My boys were nowhere to be seen. Just me, the flashes of swallows, the quiet settling of lengthening shadow, I was content. I had no need to travel to Walden's Pond to find the contemplative pleasures Thoreau describes, I could create my own pond anywhere. And that meadow in the Picos de Europa was the metaphorical pond I chose.

"Whatever is there to do all those weeks?" Friends in England asked, clearly mystified by my answer, "I'm learning to do nothing.

Bloody hard, though. It took me three weeks of watch-checking and kicking my heels on the village wall to finally be still."

Somehow it has taken me longer to find my quiet place, my pond, here in the desert of New Mexico. The summers too hot, the winter winds too bitter, the earth too littered with cactus spines and thorny goat-heads to spike me, and the no-see-um bugs too numerous I can't stay outdoors for long. Short spells, yes. Walks along the arroyos where the crunch of boots beat time to the thresher's song; and a climb to my favorite perch in the cranny of the hog back above our land where a solitary raven calls to visit.

However my challenge is to find a balance between my want of the simple quiet, against the daily chaos and my duty. Slowing down is easier said than done. Also to change my attitude.

This very June, a smiling Indian Saint, *Amma*, came to town. I'd looked forward to her visit for months. I'd not seen her for three years. Oh, so desperately I wanted her hug, a top-up to the hugs I received other years, and to experience again her gift of unconditional love.

I needed a boost to help with my caregiving. Help me with David. Too often I feel bereft of love. And yearn to be comforted, for someone to squeeze the breath out of me.

"I can't do it. I can't go it alone. Please give me strength. Please help me. I so want to be a better and loving caregiver," I prayed silently, my eyes fixed on the Saint.

I'd already stood in line for close on two hours, then a further three for my number to come up, for my turn to mount the stairs to the stage where she sat, for my turn to kneel at her feet and bury my face in her sari.

As she pulled me into her arms she looked into my eyes and laughed, and I knew without doubt I was loved, and everything was right.

Although it feels like a roller coaster now, life will calm down.

Yes, just as the fortune cookie foretold, because I became quiet inside, it had.

June 24, 2017

34. testing... testing...

Every second Thursday of the month, a group we call Nickel Stories meets to read five minutes of prose aloud. This month with barely time to drop David home, I jump back in the car and head to town for the second time that day.

I snatched up a 600-word piece called Lies Streaming. Written seven years ago, I'd all but forgotten the trip David and I took into the New Mexican Wilderness.

Re-reading my words brought back those steamy first years of our relationship, those days we hungered to be alone. But as I heard aloud the story I was reading, it came to me Parkinson's is a test of our relationship just as our trip was then.

After the initial shock of David's Parkinson's diagnosis, I decided not, that's right N-O-T to read up on symptoms ahead of time, but to face whatever presented itself as it came along. Who knew after all, and I most certainly had no idea, how David's symptoms might manifest and what speed they'd accelerate.

"You should read up on Parkinson's, know what to expect," friends insisted shaking their heads knowingly.

"Lord. No," was my answer. "Moving one problem pebble out off the path at a time I can do… less daunting than pitting my strength against a massive boulder." I spoke in a metaphor as a way of distancing myself—okay, okay, I admit it—from reality.

They just didn't get it. My way of coping. Little by little, Small things like help standing — easy. Taking over bill-paying — a pain. Giving up mountain hiking and hunting for chanterelles — too bad, but not worth fussing over. Not so easy to surmount — the most recent problem swinging his legs into bed. David's body has forgotten how, and I can barely lift them.

"... just another problem to solve, darling," I rave panting. "We'll find a way."

Seeing our lives as a test has given me a new perspective. Wow. If our relationship can survive Parkinson's perhaps we'll score an A grade, or at the very least a pass. I saw again my school reports, hung my head as each subject was read out.

Could do better... Sloppy work... If she put her mind to it... This girl has no background in this subject."

Oh the hopeless shame of it. Labeled dumb, I gave up on algebra, trigonometry and Latin right then and daydreamed my way through classes that sent me to asleep. Wasted years. Couldn't the head teacher understand my schooling had been experiential?

I knew and had experienced mysteries my English peers had never seen: an elephant felling a teak tree, a mighty Tusker caparisoned in red and gold bearing a bridegroom to his bride; a muzzled dancing bear, a beggar child, and a circus girl my age, each enslaved to earn their keep.

I heard and understood the temple bells and calls to prayer. I spoke Hindi as a child. I rode a pony to school in the Kashmiri Himalayas, and once rode hundreds of scary miles balanced on wooden planks across the flooded plains of the swollen Jamu River. Inhaling the scents of an ancient and living civilization my schooling took place far beyond the four walls of a classroom.

Without the teachings of the Spiritual Path I've followed these past thirty years I could not have even sat the test David and I are now sitting. I'd have crumpled long ago.

People are always asking, "How do you do it?"

My answer, "I just do," and shrug. "We have to."

But inside I know loving David with his Parkinson's and my strug-gle to cope is just a tiny part of a picture, which, being earthbound and of which we have no understanding, I believe whatever David and I do is perfect for us. Perfect in the sense there is always some-thing to learn from everything happening to us.

Good. Bad. Joyful. Sad.

Days when David's slowness has me tapping my feet are my opportunity to learn a little patience. To slow down. A lesson in acceptance.

"Surely moving David safely is more important than speed," I chastise myself. "Really, get a grip. Who cares if we're two minutes late?"

I do. You must understand I have a hang-up about being late. Suffer a near anxiety attack when I'm not on time, Lesson for him. Lesson for me.

Sometimes David droops so sad I drop everything and rush to hug and smother him with kisses. It's natural now, but wasn't always, for until the age of fourteen I'd forgotten how to love. I had to re-learn how to give and receive the love I'd not experienced since I was a toddler in my Ayah's arms.

I'd shut down, you see when I was snatched from my mother in India and taken form all I knew to a country across the black water, the English called "Home."

Not a sob story, but an explanation why being demonstrative is so hard.

I was teen before love re-surged. Then later with my children, when they were born and became my teachers. Now David is my teacher.

"Ah, this is how love feels. Now I remember." I hug him.

*　　*　　*

So here, the story of our first weekend away together that I read before the prose group.

LIES STREAMING

I'm not a liar by nature so I was sort of shocked to hear myself telling such a whopper. Even as the lie tumbled from me, I flinched aware I was lying. I had never actually assembled that particular tent – the one I'd bought in a garage sale a few weeks back, "Oh yes. It's easy," I'd sworn in answer to my new boyfriend's questioning.

"Do you know how to put up this tent? But THIS tent, have you put THIS tent up before?" He pressed.

Wanting to please him, I nodded blithely hoping a nod did not qualify as a lie.

"A tent's a tent, after all," I convinced myself. "Couldn't be too difficult to fathom."

The navy blue tent looked no different from the dome tent I, and my husband-once-removed, had put up in Spain years before – apart from the color that is, which had glowed a shocking orange.

We, my new boyfriend and me, were at that point in our relationship of putting ourselves in all kinds of situations to discover how un or how com – patible we were.

We'd survived many road trips, and drove two and a half days over the border to San Miguel de Allende, marveled at the Monarch butterflies forming a trembling pyramid over the tree, and bathed naked in an underground hot spring lit by a beam of moonlight through the rock's fissure.

But now the time had come for the big test. A camping test, which I discovered AFTER, sounds more romantic than it is.

In our case, we packed the car and drove to Canyon de Chelly singing.

We settled for isolated campground where the tent site was positioned on a pancake-flat patch of dirt.

"Perfect," I declared.

"And close to a cluster of Rabbit Bush to pee behind," we giggled, for we were still cheerful at that point.

Stretching and pegging the rectangle of ground sheet we laid the nylon fly to face the rising sun. Next we lined up the tent poles in neat rows. So far so good. Time came to snap the sectioned rods straight and insert them through the loops of the dome and fit their ends one into the other — well that is what should have happened, because by then I was wishing they'd been numbered, the poles I mean, and I remembered to bring a copy of the 1–2–3 instructions.

David was a big man, sort of like Popeye after he's consumed a mound of spinach, but however forcefully we tried, my trial fiancé with all his strength failed to pop the pole ends into their slots. It became obvious the poles had grown too long and dark was fast descending.

One look at his face and I knew I'd better do something and fast to unclamp his hard set lips. Come up with a plan that second to avoid the looming catastrophe I could see, but had not yet quite fallen, if you get my meaning.

Quick as a flash, I snapped open a folding chair, faced it towards the setting sun, back towards me, and thrust a neat chigger of Tequila in his hands crooning calmly as I could, "Here, sit here. Relax. I'll get the damn thing up, no worries."

With neither his strength nor any notion of what to do, criss-crossing the free ends of the poles into a bundle, I lashed them together like lodge-poles of a teepee, which made the inside a little strange considering it was supposed to a dome tent. Round. No matter. The damn thing was up. That's all I cared. And after a couple of stiff margaritas, my boyfriend didn't give a toss either.

We only camped that one night. Next day we checked into a motel.

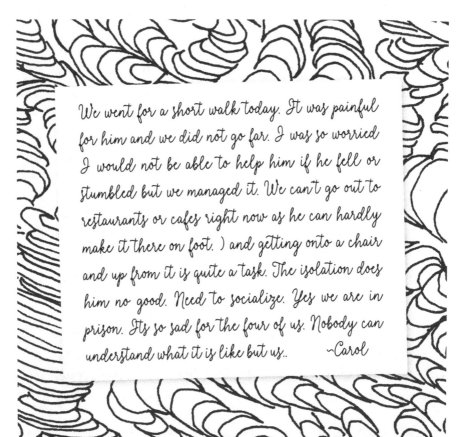

We went for a short walk today. It was painful for him and we did not go far. I was so worried I would not be able to help him if he fell or stumbled but we managed it. We can't go out to restaurants or cafes right now as he can hardly make it there on foot.) and getting onto a chair and up from it is quite a task. The isolation does him no good. Need to socialize. Yes we are in prison. Its so sad for the four of us. Nobody can understand what it is like but us.. ~Carol

35. a bird's eye view

The high dry temperatures of New Mexico have burned for over a week. Smoke from a wild fire blazes thirty miles south driving us indoors. Curtains pulled, the whirring fans do little more than stir the air and flap the hems of the living room curtains. Semi-comatose I answer the phone.

"Can you come to stay? I'm having a week-long open house, a family reunion for my mother's side of the family," It was David's young cousin. "Love for you to meet them and see my property."

An escape to his cabin in the higher Colorado elevation for a few days? We could hardly wait.

When he first bought the river property six months back, we'd oo-hed and aahed over photos of the land and his tales of wandering elk. His first home ever apart from a yurt in Hawaii, Yes. Yes. Yes, of course we wanted to see for ourselves.

The three hour drive was easy, but finding his place... ?

Out of phone range, no GPS contact, Siri fell mute, and from the hazy directions floating somewhere inside my head, realized I'd missed the correct turn by miles.

"What to do, David?" I'd croaked almost in tears.

Our Highlander idled in the middle of a dirt-packed lane. No houses, no traffic, no promised landmark red roof or tan cabin that I could see — nothing, unless cows and horses count.

But like Siri, David kept silent. His head stayed slumped.

"I've had it. One more try and I'm giving up and checking us into the nearest motel." I thumped the steering wheel and hung a U-ey.

Backtracking five miles, the tan cabin suddenly rose from a meadow on the left and on its gate hung a sign.

"Welcome David and Liz." I wanted to kiss the ground with sheer relief.

His cousin waved us into his drive. Dogs barked and the house spilled people as we drove up — his mother, sister, aunts, cousins, and friends, only two of whom David recognized.

Clearly occupied, a motor home from Arizona trailed an electric cable to the garage. I heard an a/c humming from inside.

"Hi." A young man in shorts greeted poking charcoal embers in a half oil drum… three women in the kitchen happily chatting prepped veggies for the barbecue… a grey haired man clutching a beer bottle sprawled bare foot on the magazine littered sofa, and the women sitting with him raised their glasses to us as we were introduced.

David's cousin, our host, and his sister brought two extra cushions for David's chair, handed him a coke, and me a glass of Rosé. My spirits rose as they made us feel at home.

"Now you are whose cousin?" "You belong to whom?" We never quite resolved the mystery during our two days there.

Dusk settling and still rattled from the drive, I kicked off my shoes and walked onto the deck. Oh God did I want to breathe. Bury the hellish upset in solitude. I needed a few minutes alone.

The air outside brushed softly cool. Dusk hovered before slowly dropping without a sound.

As I stood there looking, listening, a small bird flew across the field below me, folded its wings and plunged into the knee-high field grasses. As if on cue, a pair of long-legged herons winged overhead following the riverbed flowing from the distant Navajo Peaks. Every direction I turned the land stretched a paradise of green and tumbling water pocketed with shadowed trout pools.

"Tomorrow," I promised myself shivering in anticipation. "I'll take a dip however icy." And when I did next day, and slipped into a pool sheltered by hazel and willow trees, I emerged as a newborn smoothed and worry-free as I had years back from the Himalayan snow waters of the Ganges at Rishikesh.

"Dinner, everybody." David's cousin called us to the table on the deck, and settled David upright in the chair beside me.

"Thank you all. It's wonderful having all of you here," *Kind-host* toasted.

Glasses lifted and the feast began. This was how living should be.

I looked around at the ring of faces lit by solar fairy lights and stars, observed the easy flow of conversation, the quick banter, rapid passing of dishes and serving and eating, and remembered normal.

The *normal* David and I had long forgotten and could never be again. Outsiders — that's what we'd become, I realized suddenly sad. Don't get me wrong. Not one of the group minded the dropped food and messed up place, and jumped to spoil and fuss over David whenever they could.

I'd taken but a mouthful of salmon when I became aware the table fell suddenly quiet-all eyes fixed on David.

Someone nudged me pointing wordlessly in his direction. I looked over. Nothing unusual as far as I could tell. As always he sat hunched over and tilted sideways with his face just inches from his plate. His fork lay in his hand.

"What? What?" It took me a minute. Then I got it. They were seeing him keeled over for the first time and were concerned. Alarmed even. His posture, silence and slowness, the child's manner of his eating — odd. Disturbing.

As I swapped places with his cousin, to better load food into David's fork the people around the table deliberately turned to talk among themselves to hide their own discomfort and to protect David from the perceived humiliation of being fed.

Not David. He showed no such embarrassment. Unperturbed, passive, eyes shut, allowing me to feed him, he sat opening his mouth for the next tidbit like a baby bird. No bother to me, but I became aware our presence—the very act of not staring cost effort.

It takes a camera lens, a magnifying glass, to expose flaws we no longer notice. In my case, it took immersion into a healthy group of people to show me how handicapped David has become, and how aberrant our interactions. Some might say dysfunctional.

We're a peculiar sight, I don't deny — two grown-ups acting as we do — enmeshed, symbiotic, as Siamese twins.

At our first supper in Colorado, the theatre of that single meal, the bird's eye view of how our actions appeared to other people shocked. The sight of my feeding David, for example, cutting the food on his plate, tipping up his elbow to drink, responding for him when he's switched off, guiding his hands for the arms of the chair before he sits, me walking backwards, pulling David by his hands to get him to the table.

I'm so used to the way we are now, me doing for David what he can't, I'd never seen what others see, seeing us for the first time.

Disruptors, oddballs aptly describe us, the couple I viewed from above. Like the naked king in the nursery story of the King's new clothes, however normally we are treated, regular we are not.

I imagine all we caregiving partners feel the same.

I mean, how often have I come across a person slumped seemingly unresponsive in a restaurant? Excepting David, Never is my answer. And if I did, I'm sure I'd panic believing he'd suffered a stroke and call 911.

I shy away from the image. I feel a creeping guilt for putting David in such awkward situations. Not fair to David. Not fair to fellow diners. I'm at a tipping point. Whether to struggle on hoping David will survive the meal awake, or should give in and accept it's plain stupid of me to expect he will. The selfish side of me hungers to eat out, visit friends and keep on playing normal. Refuses to be a stay-at-home.

I'm just not ready.

Back to my bird's-eye-view:

I imagine myself a stranger seeing us for the first time, observe an elderly couple; a harried caregiver with wild eyes protective of her husband, and a shuffling, bent wreck of a man, handicapped by some crippling affliction, clinging to his wife's arm.

"Woah," I thought taken aback. "Without my noticing I've become the woman crossing the Senior Center parking lot I described in my first blog. Wispy haired, downtrodden, a frump."

In just a year, I've—we've—changed that much? From my imaginary perch on the treetop I take a good hard look. Don't much like what I see.

Gone the sparky, the full-of-bounce person I used to be, the person, who only a few years back, would have thrown her clothes to the wind and rushed into the icy water laughing and splashing and calling pussy-foot to David for not joining me.

A few more sun-spots, wrinkles, aches and pains, and age related stiffness, not too bad for my years, those I can live with. But who the hell is that foot-stamping woman prone to stressed-induced outbursts so deeply exhausted she can barely smile?

Go sit down. Get your hair cut. Put on some lipstick. Get a grip, woman, I wanted to cry. *You should see yourself.*

Innocent and brutally honest, out of the mouths of babes and...

"Are you poorly, Grandpa?" asked my four-year-old grandson studying David's face and hands when David's tremor first signaled his Parkinson's.

Looking down at his hands, he began shaking his own limbs — not in mimicry, but trying to understand how trembling felt. Adults politely avoid commenting. Not so a child.

Today there is no escape, like my four-year-old grandson I am seeing the truth of how things really are.

*　　*　　*

I can hear the stars tonight
he said sitting on the edge of our bed
was it only yesterday he whispered his midnight words
and laying back beside me pulled the milky-way
through the open window his face beautiful
a poem beside me on my pillow?

today
I cup my hands
press my face into the grey-green waters of his world
feel his fingers clamp about my wrists to keep from drowning
treading water clinched as one we struggle
in the raging waves of his Parkinsonian sea
to reclaim the kingdom he once ruled
hold on my love I'm here I cry

flotsam
my voice bubbles upwards to the surface
I cannot hold him and watch him sink beyond my reach

*　　*　　*

July 8, 2017

36. crossroads

The fantasy of normality vanished last week. David's mind slipped one brief moment.

"Ma. Ma." I heard him call.

Was he hallucinating? Could he mean me? My breathing stopped.

"Mum. Mum. Are you there Mum? I'd like some water please." Persistent, he pleaded again.

Was this the beginning of the end? The part of the story where the husband no longer knows his wife? And the wife's husband sinks from sight? Brutal as a blow from a wooden club, David's words struck with an agony I can't describe.

"So what he called you Mum?" A friend I'd confided in retorted, "It's nothing but a muddling of age. My own mother often called me mother the last year of her life."

I listened to her rabbit on. Justify her deceased mother's ramblings.

"It's natural," she continued. "Makes total sense he sees you as his mother as you're doing motherly things." She looked at me. "Nothing to get upset about. It's not as though he's trying to be hurtful."

No slip of the tongue, I saw David calling me mother as a momentous marker. I covered my face. She clearly had no notion of the distress I felt.

David and I stood shivering on the Parkinson's-swept landscape at a lonely crossroads. Behind us the hill we'd struggled to climb. Before us the signpost.

Caution DEAD END. NO EXIT. Its single arm pointed downhill.

As David's *wife-care-giver-partner-lover-friend*, watching Parkinson's relentless grip pull him slowly, oh so cruelly slowly underwater tortures me. The increasing episodes when his eyes dull, and his grip on reality loosens, I feel his hold on life release.

How can we, us helpless observers, bear the incremental fading away of our loved one, caregivers? How can I ease his and my distress?

Too difficult for me to verbalize my sadness, I penned the poem instead — the one included at the beginning of this week's blog post.

More and more frequently these days, I catch his stare, eyes wide and wild as if he no longer knows what is going on. Where he is.

"Are you okay? Does the world sometimes seem confused, darling?" I ask.

"Yes. Often. I'm deteriorating," David admitted quietly, his voice a monotone.

"How can I help?" I asked rubbing the back of his neck. "What can I can do to make it easier?"

My heart clenched. I half expected him to say he was ready to seek out a place where medically assisted suicide is legal.

"I'll just have to allow things to run their course." His words surprised me.

Though our arms were about eachother, our eyes, lowered, didn't meet.

What is there but pain to see in his eyes after all? The flat resignation of knowing his condition is gathering speed and sweeping him faster and faster towards his end. The weakening of his will to keep on living.

The eyes of my stepmother's ancient and sick cat held that same hopelessness of surrender to the inevitable as she was carried away to be euthanized.

So too the chicken my sons tethered to their tent pole while deciding how to deal with the poor thing. They'd won the live bird at the annual village Fiesta of Waiters in Spain. Accepting its certain death, it molted one dulled plume at a time till the owner of the local bar put the poor creature out of its misery.

And a human being? In all but three states of this civilized country, America, death by choice is not an option. A human must endure, however great his suffering.

What more is there to say about our tragedy?

David is acutely aware of the path ahead. Knows I know its destination too. Dwelling on such helps neither one of us. Nor does collapsing crumpled into a moaning heap.

The only way to live is to try and focus on what we can, not what we cannot do. But the effort costs David his last ounce of willpower. My watching his struggle costs too.

I've always been myself even when I was not myself, declaimed Mad King George in the film we were watching. Turns out the poor man wasn't mad but suffering a neurological disease which turned his behavior and mind on end.

David turned to me.

"I feel like that... that I am *myself...* even when I can't move or speak."

So very brave, his confession made me weep.

That evening sharing cocktail hour — his, a virgin Bloody Mary, a full-blown one for me — I picked the conversational thread where we'd left off that morning. I wanted, needed, answers.

The time had come for me to stand back and take a long cold look at David's turbulent disease. Check and draw up a list of what Parkinson's had robbed my David. Skills he once was proud of but has no more. The love of hiking we shared — striding Hamilton Mesa in the Pecos Wilderness, our barefoot wandering White Sands National Monument in southern New Mexico, and the tropical beaches and wild places the world over.

Can't say the same for his fine motor skills. Apart from the delicate watercolors he used to so beautifully to mix and compose, I tease he's an all-thumbs man. We laughed remembering how as an intern sewing up a wound, the nurse reached for his needle.

"Would you like me to take over, doc?" She stared horrified at the clumsy repair.

Short term memory of the *what's-the-hell's-his-name* variety, well, that's a plague for both of us. Word-finding too.

What is new though, is the dimming of David's verbal comprehension. Simple action phrases such as take a step back, sideways, forwards, though repeated everyday, more and more often leave him frozen. Quizzical.

"Put your teeth in," I might say pushing the uppers inside his mouth. I turn away for a second to find the damn gnashers are out and swimming in his tooth mug once again.

These days I take more effort to be more aware of his confused state. Spell out the whens and wherefores of we're going, what we're doing, what it is I'm asking him to do.

Tapping the limb, using gesture I translate my words for him imagining how would be if I were shipwrecked on an island where people spoke an alien language as happened to poor Cabeza de Baca in the 1500s. Never forgot that film. The trauma he went through trying to decipher the tribal lord's jumbled sounds.

We're off to France in two weeks and I've already two bags packed pack. David harried me to sort his clothes believing we left in a few days. Today, tomorrow, a week or a day, time is no longer measured as before.

In the hopes of preventing a pre-travel panic attack as he did last year the night before we flew I'm trying out a homeopathic remedy.

Don't think I can cope if he *throws a wobbly* again. And to help him understand where we're flying to and when.

I've decided to involve him more in the actual choosing of shoes and shirts and the packing of what he calls sleeping T-shirts. Yesterday we sat in the living room checking passports, tickets and itinerary.

David held each document satisfying himself I had the correct dates and times. Confession. I've been known to turn up for a flight to find I'm either a day early or, shame on me, two days late.

Time for this caregiver to have a minder of her own.

"Do you ever forget my name?" I gripped the fingers of my left hand steeling myself for his answer.

"Not usually." His hesitation told a different story.

"So who am I, darling?" I pressed.

"You're Liz. You're my darling wife." He turns toward me.

We smile at one another. Grateful. Thankful we are still husband and wife.

David is back.

I had never read a blog until, for no good reason, I clicked on yours. I am truly sorry to see what you and David are coping with at a time in life when things should be simple and lovely. My 40 years as a Neurosurgeon provided me with much exposure to neurological disability. Your blog had given me a better understanding of the depth of the problems for the solo caregiver. ~MJ.

July 15, 2017

37. madam your slip is showing

"Chr***t is that you?" A friend I'd not seen for half a year accosted me in the heart clinic's parking lot. "What's going on?" She quizzed. "I hardly recognized you. You look absolutely whacked out."

Honest maybe, her greeting me that way, but not exactly uplifting after taking a Heart Stress Test. I crumpled, crushed.

Wondered if I really looked so changed. Wondered if my body was really packing up.

In truth I'd been aware the old me hung in desiccated shreds barely concealed by a fast thinning veneer of cheer. What I hadn't recognized though, was caregiving stamped its stress signature of lines across my forehead.

The plain hard physical work of the daily bodily haulings and heavings, and uppings and downings, and spoonings and dressings and washings and shavings, pill sortings and drivings to this appointment and that, gnawed at the very marrow of both my inner and outer being cutting lines deeper than those I'd earned by advancing age.

I was too down to argue. I knew she was right. Sitting back in the car, I turned the driver's mirror and saw a face leached of joy.

Orange is the new Black. The meaning of this strange phrase became suddenly clear. Old Mother Hubbard who lived in a cupboard was the new me. Old me was no more.

For the past two, or it three years now, friends warned, "Watch out. You'll collapse. Make yourself ill if you don't take care of yourself and get some help. And where would David be then?"

Yeah. Yeah. I'd shrug. Until now that is when my heart misses a beat and gives a series of arrhythmic thumps — something I previously thought of as poetic literature. But a heart missing a beat is physical I've discovered. An unpleasant manifestation of stress I don't much like. So tough as I think I am, maybe it's happening — I'm unraveling. Physically. Emotionally.

"Too much. Too much. I can't cope," I often exclaim out loud to the four walls.

I've never been a crybaby, or had massive temper tantrums before I became a caregiver. Prided myself on my inner calm, and being able to keep a hold on my mind thanks to my meditation practice. Wow. If only… I could command my emotions as I could then.

Increasingly, my frequent outbursts shock David. Shock me.

"It's okay," I reach to comfort him as he reaches to comfort me.

Poor man. He looks at me as if I'm a brittle papyrus scroll. American and Psychiatrist that he is, he turns solemn, says, "You need to talk to someone."

"Better out than in. Crying's a healthy outlet, and I'm just tiredW," I sob. "… so tired, that's all."

And it really is. Healthy, I mean. Well, if ones crying is occasional.

Better than venting to my long-suffering friends, or seeking out a therapist, I make an appointment to luxuriate in a hot-stone massage with a friend I've known for thirty years and then take the two if us out to lunch. Oh, I was looking forward to my day. Oh, so ready.

But the planned morning turned into one from hell. The money transfer arranged ten days back hadn't happened throwing our account into the red with no funds to buy euros for next week's trip to France. "Cancelled," the teller sneered.

On top of that, David's sitter didn't turn up and couldn't be reached... David's drug prescription hadn't been filled... the optometrist refused issue the correct eyeglass prescription... the hearing aid clinic was closed... Siri, deaf to my bidding, wouldn't dial a single number for me.

Thrown into chaos, no damn help anywhere, I wept defeatist, useless tears, collected David, canceled my massage, canceled my lunch date, and headed for home to bury my face in the pillow.

All silly annoyances of daily life I'd have laughed off even a year or two ago, now loomed as insurmountable as Everest.

In my distress it came to me, the course I'd once taken on keeping one's cool, one's concentration. And how in the mid-quiet of meditation, sudden bursts of revving motorcycles, followed by bouts of coughing interrupted to test my inner calm right at the moment I sank deep within. No problem then, the sounds buzzed no more bothersome than a distant fly. But now... the smallest upset... and I splatter.

"What the hell has happened to me?" I groaned.

"You're in flight or fight mode by necessity," a friend replied. "Running on adrenaline?"

"I used to smile," I answered downcast. Saw a vessel empty of the person who resided there back when. Once, twice and then again last week, the same warnings about cracking up seemed to hound me.

"By the by did you know an enormous percentage of caregivers die before the person they are caring for? And as for those caregivers over seventy... well... " chirped a woman sharing my lunch table at the Senior Center, staring hard at me.

So how is it I've hardly a grey hair on my head? And why it's not shocked white with all the heart-stopping accidents happening?

At every thump, and crash as David hits the floor I fly to locate him in dread I'll find him badly injured or stone dead. Nearly came true last Sunday.

Nothing unusual. David alone for an hour. A weekly pattern: the program, David in his chair, sitting safely, content watching the telly's Sunday Morning and Face the Nation show on his own.

Confession. I was late. Twenty minutes later than usual.

Returning from a mornings writing session with a friend, my head running with all manner of things to share, I was tripping up the path when loud clapping startled me. Confused, I scoured the yard. Spotted him... David stretched straight out on the hot stones face up to the scalding sun redder than a Red Racer snake.

Oh God the shock — David so burned. So still. I'm normally calm in a crisis. Not that one. I raced to him whimpering, "Oh. Oh David, David. Are you hurt? Can you move? What happened? How long have you been here? I'm calling 911."

"No. Water. Water," David gasped.

Throwing my papers and sunglasses to the ground I sped to the house for something to shade his face... hat... umbrella... Backwards and forwards I ran crying aloud, "What to do. What to do? Too heavy. Too heavy, I can't move you, darling. I'm calling 911."

"No. No. "Get our tenant." David reiterated.

So I took off... ran for a drinking straw, ran for his mug, ran for the tenant, thumping his door, bursting it open half sobbing and yelling, "Oh, oh, oh. Quickly. I need help," and without stopping for his answer circled back to be with David.

Legs, heart, thoughts pounding, I took off to grab the outdoor cushions, one for his head, two beside him to roll onto. Our tenant appeared. Calm. He coped. Squeezed my shoulder. Comforted.

"First let's get him up." Deadweight though he was, somehow the two of us managed to heave him up and into a wheelchair. Out of breath, heart pounding, my limbs jellied. But for the Emergency Responder on the line, keeping me together until the crew arrived I'd have collapsed.

Iced cloths, rehydration and a little oxygen later David revived enough to refuse a trip to hospital. Glad he did. Though legs, face scalp and thighs glowed cockscomb scarlet he somehow escaped serious heatstroke and never blistered.

Visions flash… the what ifs… burnt eyeballs if his spectacles hadn't gone flying as he fell… the fiery concentration of sunbeams… third degree burns… imagining David's ordeal makes me queasy.

The point of telling this story is the incident manifested itself a day later with a painful four days of colitis forcing me to admit I'm vulnerable and human. Yup. Time to recognize my slip is showing. Admit to feeling my body and my mind bend to the daily blast of caregiving.

I am as a Saharan dune re-shaped by the desert winds one grain at a time.

On the drive last week to Albuquerque, captivated by the green-ing of the desert landscape after last week's torrential rains, I was intrigued by a tangle of interwoven wagon tracks, pale and beige, wending up the hill towards a gap in the otherwise straight ridge-line. Eroded by centuries of plodding feet and hooves and the grinding wheels of pioneers, the pass to the Rio Grande valley lay thirty feet below the skyline.

Only a traveler journeying for a second time would recall how the pass looked before man's be-spoiling. So too, David, my family, my friends, only they notice the deepening cracks etched in my person.

July 22, 2017

38. if only caregiving was always...

Stepping from the airport shuttle at Albuquerque Sunport's curb-side, the desk clerk summoned a wheelchair and checked in the two of us, overstuffed bags and all. Right there. No fuss no lines. No dragging cases to the Check-in desk inside. As he took each bag, weighed and placed them on the moving belt I felt the caregiver's mantle round me flutter then let slip. Pouffe... bags and mantle vanished from my sight. Just like that.

"You'll next see your suitcases in Geneva," he smiled handing me our boarding passes.

L-I-B-E-R-A-T-I-O-N.

Unburdened, I stood a moment and allowed myself to stretch.

"Ah, this is how it is to be a regular person again," I sighed looking round the hall of milling passengers.

I'd forgotten how glorious was the feeling of walking free. I swung my lime-green Bagini for the sheer joy of not having David's dead weight clinging to my arm.

Like our bags, David and his wheelchair disappeared from sight through Security and out. I trotted to catch up. Half-heartedly, I confess.

My own person, at my own pace I paused at a gift shop not because I wanted to buy any of their stuff but because my hands were duty-free to finger the fridge magnets depicting what tourists to New Mexico are expected to like: a Roadrunner, a sun Zia symbol, a string of chile-peppers, a Jackalope, and the ubiquitous howling coyote in a cowboy neckscarf.

From there on, the journey unrolled like the Indian bedding roll I'd traveled with as a child. Waiting at the gate to board, I could almost smell the spice of curries cooking, hear the chai-wallah calling, see the groups of Indian families bedded on the station platform beside us, my mother, brother and me, waiting as we waited for the blackened steam engine to manifest from the dark.

Yes, travel was romantic then. Adventurous too.

"We'll begin with pre-board," the announcement landed me back in Albuquerque.

Safely and comfortably settled, at last the plane lifted us into the vacuum of the unknown. No routine to follow, no appointments to keep, no phones to answer, this was the life.

From the aisle window I watched Salt Lake spread low and flat like buttered bread below the peaks and ridges of the Wasatch mountains.

"We're on holiday, my sweetie-pie. We're going to have a lovely time," I patted David's hand, my mind and body sighing their agreement and relief.

David turned his head to me, nodded, munched a cookie then slept. An hour flashed and the flight was over.

Airport assistance equals wheelchair. I call them airport angels. Always happy, smiling full of chat the chair-pushers magically appear to meet the plane, and whisk David to the connecting gate.

For once it's not me who humps David's heavy frame. Not me who steadies his balance. Not me who carries his bags. I'm once again his companion. Once more his wife. That's what I mean when I say I wish caregiving were always as easy.

For the weeks before travel I squirrel away a stash of fives, tens, and one dollar bills to parcel out in grateful thank-yous. Sort of like dealing cards.

With time enough to do all he needed in order to avoid a trip to the plane's toilet cubicle during the nine-hour flight to Amsterdam, we exited the Family restroom relieved.

The travel-tip I have to offer anyone traveling with a mobility-compromised and incontinent companion is *dress in layers:* I'm speaking undergarments beneath trousers. Three pairs to be precise. Cut and rejoin the sides of the two inner pairs with duct-tape. Peel off the tape for easy removal without undressing and... *Ta-dah... Voilà...* with a yank and sleight of hand as fast as a magician's, a dry pair lays next to skin. No struggle needed to remove shoes and pants. No fear of embarrassing leaks.

Airport-angel jumped the line of waiting passengers and in a minute strapped us comfortably in the airbus bound for Amsterdam.

The airhostess taking over my caregiving duties, fussed and tended David, ensured his legs were elevated, his head cradled by a pillow, and a drink within reach. Redundant and needed only as an overseer of David's care I ordered a Scotch. David did likewise. I watched him while he ate his fish course, then dig his spoon into a cream slathered chocolate dessert, and order a port.

"Bodes well," I thought to myself foreseeing five weeks of family holiday ahead and slept blissfully for four hours straight. Morning broke, the lights flipped on. Breakfast appeared and was cleared, away, and with just one bump we were back on earth.

One connecting flight remained. David was pretty well done for. But thanks to our Airport-angel we even made a bathroom stop. Whacked out and jet-lagged the last hop to Geneva passed in a daze. Deplaning David turned into a two-man job... first plane seat into the aisle wheelchair, from aisle chair to a regular sized one for the speed ride through immigration and customs.

All at once we were expelled into Arrivals with our feet firm on French soil.

Oh, the joyful hugs and kisses of welcome as the family gathered round and loaded David, bags et moi into the car for the forty minute ride to their farmhouse.

So here I am in the mountains breathing in the soft air, and gazing at the jagged peaks of the French Alps rising from our bedroom window. Here I am where the burdens of caregiving break manageable, scatter like the red roofs of Mont Saxonnex's tiny village.

I stepped back. The family took over.

"Let me help, Grandpa. This leg David. Move this one. Bend your knee. Hold here. Now push. Up. Well done," congratulates the six year old.

I suppose this is the way aging and elder care used to be. Family stepping in, keeping Grandma, grandpa with them at home. David. Me. And they have offered. My daughter-in-law and son.

"The ground floor apartment is yours whenever you say the word." Mean it too. No question of being stuffed away in some institution. Discarded. Branded useless just because we're old Makes me, us, feel safe just knowing.

Small is Beautiful, wrote Schumacher.

The village in Spain's Picos de Europa where we summered for eleven years was living proof. I remember the elderly... Angel, the blind man with his stick perched all day long on the village wall. "Hola. Hola Senor Angel," the villagers greet as they pass him by.

Then there was Antonia, mother of Juan the owner of the Bar *Juanon*, incontinent and disorientated from Alzheimer's, treated respectfully by any villager encountering her and gently escorted home. Same for Mario, an autistic and developmentally delayed young man obsessed with a length of string before his eyes. No question of shutting him away, he spent his life happy at his mother's side.

I remember watching him swaying at the field's edge in the corn stubble, content, swinging his string while she scythed.

"Have you thought of putting David in a home?" People in the States continually ask.

You mean like a dog? screams my mind and felling my heart against my rib bones.

"If I were him," people persist giving me what I call the look, "I'd have chosen to *go* a long time since."

Was the insinuation I should do away with David? Be rid of my husband? Or. He should do away with himself?

I cower under the implication of their words.

"We still have many good times." Ignoring the look, their disbelief, I say. Remembering, remembering all we have, all the precious moments we share, so precious we neither of us are ready to let the other go.

Here our first night in France cozied soft in the warmth of body heat, we lie together, our pinkies curled, joining us. Reluctant to sleep.

> I miss the man who he was. When you know it, won't get any better it's a burden. I was grateful to read that you too suffer from anger, frustration, moments of madness. Sometimes I think I am such a failure but I am not. I am a careyiver and I am doing the best I possibly can   ~Carol

39. Where everything is possible

I could sprout wings and jump high as a Masai warrior competing for a bride when the sun shines and shadows bleach invisible and everything seems possible.

And here in the softer climate of France surrounded by family, happy is how I feel. It's not that I've abdicated from my caregiving role, but tending to David's needs is entirely manageable now the family has stepped in and I no longer need to shoulder the load alone.

Before David's mouth opens to a "can-you-help-me-please," my son Miles, granddaughter and eldest grandson have leapt to their feet to help him up or down from his chair.

"I've got you. Lean on me," my daughter-in-law, Kate, encourages.

David's hands clamp around her shoulders and together they inch down the twenty-one-step outdoor staircase each time we leave their farmhouse. Some days, when he's on the wobble, I follow pulling back on a yoga belt I've wrapped about his waist.

I shower and dress him of course, escort him on bathroom runs, and take my turn to fetch and carry. But oh, the heavenly bliss of relinquishing some of David's care.

Here, spun into a vortex where dishes and cutlery compete for table space. Pens, torn envelopes, tools and half repaired objects spread on last week's newspaper continually appear and disappear between mealtimes. And oh, and did I mention the revolving pile of laundry waiting to be folded? David can be the person he is, and that's a Grandpa. Sat at the head of the table, offered first choice of food, David is king.

Quiet. Grandpa's talking, and we hush and listen. However rambling his story, however groan-making his joke, we are all so pleased to hear him joining in.

David rides in the front seat of the car, too, even if the limpid green crevasse of Les Bosson's glacier below Mont Blanc goes unnoticed, thanks to his eyes being frozen shut.

And me? At last I can be Grandma, mother and mother-in law all rolled into one. I have barely lifted a finger since I've been here.

"Come," I call my grandson. "Read something to Grandpa and me in French."

"Now," my granddaughter yells. "Do as granny says," and grandson reluctantly unglues himself from the cartoon on the television screen.

Yes, in their household there is a lot of shouting. Reminds me of me. The young family I once had. The young mother I used to be.

"Anything I can do to help?" I ask, none too enthusiastically.

Perched on a kitchen stool, chatting, sampling a glass of some new wine my son and daughter-in-law discovered in a local *Cave*, a spectator, my legs elegantly crossed, I watch the evening's chaotic preparations for the evening meal. Elephant ear-sized leaves of *Blet*, Swiss chard, come under the knife and wait ready in a pan.

An ear-splitting yell hastens my grandson from the garden to hurry with the sprig of mint to add to the newly dug potatoes before they are over-cooked. Miles and Kate squabble turn-take stirring the potage.

This is how respite should be... the best way to renew. No need to stuff David into a home in order for me to recoup. Here David observes... head honcho of the family. Here I feel my energy returning.

"What, ALONE?" People query, disbelief and occasionally a tinge of disapproval in their voices. "All the way to France? How the devil can you manage security, transfers, and getting David to all those the departure gates by yourself?" They exclaim when they hear David and I are off to France on our travels.

It seems they don't get it, traveling with David is a *doddle* compared to home, thanks to wheelchairs, airport-angels, air-hostess/stewards... one to wheel him to the gate, one to tuck him into his seat. At home I am the only one around to jockey him to the starting gate for the day's tumultuous race.

If our friends just saw David's smile, saw how he is loved and welcomed, they'd understand WHY the effort, trials of flying and jetlag are worth it.

No obligations, we have more time. Lover-husband, loving-wife, time to listen to the snuffling snores as the other sleeps, time to stroll our favorite mountain road together with our grandson and the dog, and stop awhile to pluck the last of the wild raspberries from a patch we remembered from last year.

Back at the house perched on a couple of tree stumps placed to face the sun setting below us in the Chamonix valley, we sit in easy silence.

At the end of this week our 18 year-old granddaughter begins her new life in Aberdeen University, Scotland leaving her mother to a near empty-nest.

It's hard finding oneself redundant overnight... no joggins, miniskirts, backless T-s and flimsy garments tangled with the washing, and no lovely daughter with whom to huddle cheek to cheek beside binge-watching "Game of Thrones," or "Dancing With the Stars" on the computer. Mother, daughter, I see them giggle over confidences shared as only girls and women can, so I know how much she will be missed.

Suddenly bereft, as I was once, will she start talking to herself? I don't think Maggie, the ginger-haired goat delivered yesterday to board with us while her owners holiday, will cut it as a replacement

I mourn for her. Know a little of what is to come. The weight of time. The unsettled feeling of finding myself superfluous. Unsuited though I was, and never supposed to be a caregiver, now my role is parceled, shared, and half-way gone, I don't quite recognize the shell left behind... the one waiting to be re-filled.

I watch Kate's deft movements, the clean path left by the razor blade in the blue foam lathered on David's chin. My hands sit empty, useless, fingering the minutes heaped unused in my lap. Like her, I have to relearn what it is to enjoy a cuppa undisturbed, make daytime reading a guiltless habit, and to welcome unfilled days in my calendar as pleasurable.

Strange human as I am, time, the very thing I most yearn for at home in New Mexico when I'm buried exhausted beneath more tasks than I can handle, now holds my attention, hungry.

"Cheers," we'll toast on Friday. "... To your new and wonderful life." And we'll lift a glass and celebrate with a special treat of oysters on the shell from the local supermarket, and hunks of baguette spread with the cheeses of sheep and goats, perhaps her favorite *pate forestiere*, and feel a little sad knowing the next day as she boards the plane, the house will empty of her noise, and we will miss her.

I miss David the same way. Parkinson's took him from me. Gave me him back, changed.

It's my turn to thank you for your honesty. For voicing those things of which we caregivers are mortally ashamed.. Our roles reversed, your confessions help me know there is someone out there just like me. ~Liz

August 5, 2017

40. out to pasture

Like the cows of the Savoyard, I'm out to pasture, mindless, placid...
on extended holiday with nothing much to occupy me but ensuring
David eats, sleeps, is watered and happy.

Notebook open on my lap, a pen idle in my hand, words crowding to be written escape, tumble beyond reach into the high-grass
meadows where I sit, and off down the mountainside between
the red-roofs of the village to disappear somewhere into the
Chamonix Valley.

A brown and white cow turns her limpid eyes to the stump on
which we sit among clumps of purple willow herb and orange crocus. She sets the bell about her neck *a k-tink-k-tinking*. With nothing
else to interest her, I imagine our visit to be the most eventful happening in her day.

"Do open your eyes, darling," I plead wanting David to share.

"I'm looking'," he says. But his eyes remain shut.

Do sounds evoke images inside his lids? I close my eyes. Imagine I
can hear green, the color of the grass, smell chewed cud, and cows,
and feel the blaze of orange berries clustered on Rowan tree by
the shepherd's hut. David's head bows weighted by a lassitude that
comes with the disappearance of his routine. No crammed days
filled with classes, therapies, and medical appointments.

Sun and the play of a faint breeze gentle on his face, lulled by the bells of the herd grazing about us, I wonder if he is content. A family not of his own blood, borrowed lives, not our own, our identities blur.

Hampered as he is by those three stones he carries with him at all times: *PAR-KIN-SON'S,* I wonder at the cost it's taken David to travel with me here to France. Have I expected too much of him? Pushed him beyond his limit of his courage?

These past two blogs I've related only the heads-up aspect of our travels. Now is the time to spin the coin and expose the flip side. The turmoil of night becoming day, and day night, as jetlag scrambles the hours of waking and sleeping setting his poor body-clock spinning.

"Is it time to take my medication?" He asks.

I don't think the actual travel bothers him once we're on our way and in the air. Though he never grumbles, his in-built GPS struggles to remember the layout of the farmhouse from last and other years. *Wow, can it be we've been coming here to Mont Saxonnex for eleven years now?*

The strange positioning of our bed, his chair in the living room, floor rugs that ruck and slip from beneath his feet, and raised thresholds of the French doors onto the balcony.

"Take a big step, David, " as Miles guides him to breakfast on the balcony. "Hello. There you are. Now your eyes are open."

I see him struggle to locate the grab-bars in the shower stall, an unfamiliar dangling strap to raise and lower himself onto the toilet, search for the footstool he needs to mount the high vehicle, and deal with the manhandling it takes to get David seated.

Then there is his Everest.

Those twenty-one steps of uncertainty and terror awaiting him every time we leave the house, even for a turn around the garden. Does a friend of the family, Kenton Cool, a man who has summited the highest mountain in the world more times than I have fingers, does he steel himself to overcome fear such as David's each time he climbs? Do his legs tremble and sudden waves of fear buckle his knees and leave him mid-climb neither up nor down?

Miles behind, me, or Kate in front to guide his hands to the next hand rail, David moves to each precarious foothold tread by tread. Losing confidence, sometimes collapses, and it takes three of us to coax him back to his feet.

Today setting off to lunch at a local tavern in the Solison Plateau, David descended the staircase almost unaided. But returning… a different story. David's legs began trembling as our coffee appeared, signifying the meal's end.

"Are you worried about something?" I asked recognizing the sign. "Is it the steps? Are you dreading climbing the stairs?"

"Yes." His voice shook.

Exchanging glances with Kate, slipped him an anti-anxiety pill as she and I had discussed. A test. Pills his neurologist prescribed for panic attacks and just such an event. Pills, David swore never to take. But this was an emergency measure and subterfuge a necessity.

He climbed the stairs without falling to his knees. Then began muttering about lack of money, its running out, us left with empty pockets. So anxious his whole body shook.

One day last week when I was shopping, he asked Kate if she could find his funeral insurance policy.

Did he feel death waiting? See his deceased sister beckon? For over an hour, he sat so still, I feared he was no longer living.

In New Mexico our home vibrates silent. Footfalls across the terracotta tiles, the electric hum of dishwasher, telephone bell, and voices from the damnable television occasionally invade the quiet.

Here constant explosions erupt.

"9–8–7-… 2… Come up here now," and groans of "Oh, muuum… " from the 9-year old disrupt as he bangs grumpily up the stairs. Quiet lasts no longer than a breath. The dog starts up, alerts the household a hawk is circling over the chicken coop. My son rushes for a shotgun, fires a warning salvo. Sets the hens and cockerel squawking and cats running for their lives, and wasps dive-bombing

... well, what's the harm with a little exaggeration, but you get the picture. Point is, noise is not music to David's ears.

"Let's have some quiet," he hushes me at home if I talk too loudly, too long, on the phone.

For too long we've become age-set in our ways at home... diet, mealtimes, rising and going to bed at regular hours, regulated activities on particular days... predictable... caught in a rotating routine dictated by the hands of the clock.

Me who lived before caregiving, re-awakens pleased to be shaken up by a normal household. The other half retreats, screams for the peaceful order of the familiar.

Our time in France fast shrinking, reality sinks in. I see the dark shadow of my caregiver mantle loom waiting. I see this fantasy life retreating.

On Wednesday we'll be on the road. Head for England's *green and pleasant shores*. Spend time with my eldest son, Anthony, and his husband.

I take a breath, sigh unprepared. Another journey, strange places to roost along the way, then the dark Chunnel beneath the Atlantic into the great unknown before flying home.

David crouches in his chair, eyes shut from the *melee* raging about him. A surge of compassion overwhelms me. Have I been selfish? Is all this traveling too much for him?

YES, YES, I hear some of you shout.

NO, NO, go for it. Jump for everything within reach while you can, I hear you others encourage.

41. congratulations you are a winner...

… in NFPW's 2017 National Communications Contest:

Second Place : 61C Chapbook of Poetry

Entry Title: portraits: poems by e.p. rose

Hmm. Well I may be a winner but is that who I am now? What about my caregiving role? Artist? Writer? Wife? Epithets don't sit right. How and by whom will I be judged? It's David's opinion I care about… and mine… the only one important as far as I'm concerned.

Please excuse this week's cop-out blog, but I'm on the road into the unknown till Saturday, and out of cyber contact till I make it through the Chunnel from France to a Dorset cottage in Merry Old England. Have to admit I'm a little apprehensive of taking up the reins of Chief Caregiver again after so much spoiling.

Perhaps the rest here with the family will have done me good… turned me into a nicer person. I so hate myself sometimes. Feel ashamed of losing patience with such a lovely man as David.

But back to my chapbook. My poem, Digging, came to me in a dream. And to my surprise made the short list of the Bridport's Prize for Poetry. Funny really, because though I've penned some poems, I don't consider myself a poet. More of a prose writer is how I'd describe myself. Non-fiction to be exact.

DIGGING

What are you doing? I asked
I am digging for my roots
the woman whispered
will you find them buried? I persisted
of course she nodded
pointing to the Beech tree's silver trunk
they're holding up this tree
that's my home
that's me
I am the tree
she handed me her spade
pressed my hand against the bark
feel she insisted I am alive
now you dig she encouraged
turning I found myself alone

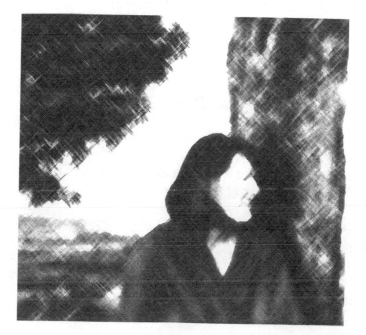

August 19, 2017

42. ...and counting

Counting kilometers, squashed beside my youngest grandson in the middle row of seats of the family car, I am riding through the countryside of France headed to England's emerald isle.

I am sad to be leaving. That the countdown has begun, for once we emerge from the Chunnel's dark tube below the English Channel, we must part. Fragment. Us, from family. Their lives. Become two. David, me, a couple isolated by continent, age and disability.

Once again: CAREGIVER : CARED. I am scared.

Wonder if my caregiver's robe will weigh too heavy for me to bear now I've tasted three weeks of a little of the cosseting I imagined old age brought.

"Sit, Stay there. I'll help David," my son, daughter-in-law, grand-children command.

And I obey, grateful I don't have to immediately struggle to my feet and tear myself from the world inside my book, thankful for this respite in my family's care.

So, as I cruise the motorway's kilometers one by one, I run my mind over the time David and I have spent together Stare through the windscreen at the signpost ahead. *CALAIS.* In a flash it is behind us. *Poof* it arrives and *poof* now it's past. *Gone.* I suppose I envy, a little, the years my young family have yet to fill.

I have so little time left in which to cram everything. With my book on Spain and my biography as one of the last babies of the Raj still to complete, paintings to paint, and the Taj Mahal to visit, I feel my future shrinking.

Here in this capsule, safe from the future, I allow myself the illusion time will cradle me forever. For a little while more I can make-believe. David and I are forever young. Supple as dolphins riding again the waves of the Indian Ocean.

So in an era where man can fly to the moon, let me dream my dream... *of a world where trees grow diamonds, and badgers weave coronets made from dragonfly wings, and my David stands tall and engages his audience of friends gathered around our dinner table with his favorite zebra in heaven joke.*

I fear my will is fading, and my strength waning and I'll no longer be able to be the sole bearer of David's care. Know I will of course. I did when David's Parkinson's was first diagnosed. Will carry the burden again. My heart freezes heavy. Remembers the effort it costs to pull off his shoes, peal off his socks, and heave his legs onto the bed and straighten his body before I'm free to drag myself into bed.

"Too old. Too brittle." These ancient bones protest.

Half an hour and we emerge the Chunnel's dark. Head for a good old British *heart-attack breakfast*. Fried eggs. Fried bacon. Fried bread. Fried Tomatoes. Fried Black pudding. Did I mention baked beans? Add those to the plate.

The family went one way. David, an old schoolfriend, and I headed south in a rented car to meet up with *always-happy-eldest-son* and his husband.

I plummeted to earth. Landed in the mire of full-on caregiving. full-on house keeping.

The thatched cottage in Dorset so picturesque and perfect by day has become for David a tangle of insurmountable stairs to climb, and lavatory seats to locate.

"Use my leg. Grip the basin here. Bend your knees. Down. Down.

Drop your arse."

Likewise to negotiate the stairs. Who would have guessed the amount of language needed to do something we most of us do without much thought.

"Hand here... Reach the banister rail... Look... See it? That's right. Now... The other hand... Grip here... Switch your weight to the other leg... Now step up... Higher... You got it... Now move it back some more to allow space for your other foot... Tha-a-a-at's it," I encourage struggling to keep my voice calm as I quell a picture of him tumbling.

I lead him with a yoga belt about his waist and keep it wound about the banister rail to stop him tumbling if he should slip. *Always-happy- eldest-son* follows. Hands at the ready to catch. "Well done," we praise. "That was your best yet."

We arrive safely. Collapse exhausted. Both dreading the repeat performance the next day. I've noticed I'm becoming the enemy in his eyes. In the bathroom mostly. He hasn't had a shower since we arrived here five days ago. I should have asked my eldest son to bathe him.

"David. David," I said yesterday finding him bent frozen halfway between standing and sitting. "I'm here to help. I'm not the enemy. Use me to support you. Feel... the arm of the chair." I entice guiding his limbs. Tap the cushioned seat.

But his eyes stayed shut till noon.

Our holiday is at its end. It's time to go home. Next Saturday's blog we'll be back in the USA to tell how we fared the journey.

If we survive.

August 26, 2017

43. re-entry burn

… otherwise known as a rude awakening.

"Bye. We'll be back for you tomorrow morning," my son, daughter-in-law, granddaughter and one grandson assured. "… with plenty of time to make the flight."

The four of them, us, kisses, hugs and chaos of bed-bouncing and handicapped amenity checking, overran the cramped space.

"Bye again. Have a good rest."

The door to our hotel room clicked shut. Alone but for a luggage cart, hotel wheelchair, our carry-ons, cases, a bag of leftover goodies from our stay in Dorset to be eaten later for our picnic supper, the sudden quiet unnerved me. I filled the electric kettle and turned to a BBC TV channel to fill the void.

"Would you like a cuppa, David, and watch the news while we re-group?"

Hunched in the wheelchair, he stared at the screen, the tea beside him growing cold.

"How about a shower, then hopping into bed?" I suggested.

Motel days when David was able-bodied and together it was the pattern we always followed.

"The bathroom's handicapped equipped and has an accessible walk-in."

David nodded he'd like that.

Damn it his eyes had shut. I let down the grab bar beside the toilet and guided his hands onto them. Neither up nor down, bum mid air, he froze. Pushing, pulling, I struggled to get him to move. No family strong arm to call, it was up to me his caregiver to get him up.

Was I nuts? Plain obstinate? I should have packed in any idea of giving him a shower but by then the two of us were naked, and I had the ridiculous notion the play of warm water would bring him back.

Once in the walk-in shower I sprayed his head and back. Shampooed his scalp. Soaped him up. He preferred standing. Clinging to the grab bars he refused to sit on the safety seat. Forget me taking a shower. I'd be lucky if I managed to get through his. Cleansing over, I held both his hands and began the slow backwards shuffle across the glistening tiles. His eyes stayed glued. Not good.

"Oh Lordy, Lordy let me reach the bathmat's safe haven, and get him into bed," I prayed silently.

"Fool. Idiot?" I cursed inwardly, while outwardly encouraging,

"Nearly there. Nearly there. Just a couple more steps, darling."

Not much of a lifeline, David, though taking baby-steps forwards, was pulling back, eyes still closed, mouth set in a grimace.

Whatever was I thinking to think I could shower him on my own?

Perhaps this was the never-again lesson I needed, for at that moment David's legs stiffened and his body slow-motioned into an unstoppable slither down the wet tiles to the floor. Landed with quite a bump. Dripping wet, David sat slumped sideways against the wall, legs turned beneath him.

Quick check: Head intact. No bleeding. No broken limbs. Thank the lord.

Comforting him I wrapped him in a towel without trying to move him.

Walked into the bedroom to devise a strategy and catch my breath.

Normally so capable, I was stumped. Should I, shouldn't I pull the emergency cord? The indignity of the two of us being found naked gave me pause. I pulled a tee shirt over his head. Pulled on my clothes in case I was forced to call for help.

Using the wheelchair as an anchor, yoga belt for leverage, and every sinew of muscle I hauled him onto his knees and from there he pushed himself to his feet. Long story short, it took over an hour to get him to bed.

Wham. Bam. Alone in the airport hotel the realization hit me. I became David's sole caregiver again. No gentle transition, no air braking burn, unlike an astronaut stepping from the dreamy confines of his spacecraft, re-entry left me stunned. My rotator cuff and back ached. My right knee screamed.

David smiled in his sleep, sheet tucked beneath his chin. Too tired to undress again, I collapsed onto my side of the bed.

Next morning, the family arrived, wheeled David and me to check-in. The airport angel appeared in the form of a supervisor to be our escort through security. I kissed and hugged our lovely family never wanting to relinquish their arms embrace.

"I miss you already," I whispered unable to stop my tears.

Would David ever see them, ever return to their French farmhouse home again? Ever visit our eldest son in England? Visit our granddaughter at Aberdeen University in Scotland, to Germany to our eldest grandson's university? Why did I live so far away?

Once in the air, wrapped in London's grey clouds, a shot of Jack Daniels in our hands, David opened his eyes, ate his ravioli and chocolate mousse un-aided. I sighed. We were safe. On our way home.

All of a sudden, David began un-clipping his seat belt. He clamped my arm.

"I must speak to someone now. We have to solve this, and get off.

This isn't right. We're doubling back."

His eyes flashed. The urgency in his voice scary.

"I'm trapped," he asserted. "I must get out of here."

If his anxiety erupted into panic we were done. What if he managed to get to his feet, made to open the airplane door, if he had to be restrained?

"Try to understand. Everything is fine, darling. We're flying home. We are in the air over Greenland and can't get off till we reach Atlanta. Then, one more little hop and we'll be in Albuquerque."

Going to Atlanta bothered him. Meant we were heading back to Heathrow.

"But why Atlanta... ?"

I pushed the button, righted his seat to upright.

"Better?" I distracted. "Oops. It's time for your pills. Now how about watching a film?"

This was an emergency situation. I slipped an anti-anxiety pill into his mouth without his say-so. Fitted his headphones. Turned on The Zoo Keeper's Wife. Prayed.

"Four hours to go. Just let him get home safely, God. I swear, I swear never to fly a long haul with him again."

Engrossed in the film, he settled for the most part. Every half hour or so he pulled off his headphones fussing we needed to get out and off. Each time I calmed him.

"Soon. We'll be landing in a few hours."

This was too hard on him. Too cruel. I realized this must be the last time I put him through such stress.

The Delta air stewards kept a kindly eye on him, helped him to sit and stand in the plane's lavatory... YES an airline with a handicapped accessible toilet... though David froze with his legs stiffened straight preventing the door from closing.

Lying there beside him, memories of life before our holiday flooded back. Time away from home so happy by contrast. How could I keep that same contentment and slow pace once we were home? And calmly accept David's limitations as the family had these past six weeks.

I shuddered at the image of who I'd become... the stressed out, shameful screecher barely able to drag through the day. Dump that unpleasant me forever, I determined.

Home. We pushed open the front door. Newly polished terracotta tiles shone unsullied as a field of standing wheat awaiting the harvester's scythe — an opportunity for us to make fresh tracks, re-structure David's last years. Mine too most likely. Nothing dramatic. Just a gradual winding down. It's not that I've given up on him. More that I've made my mind to take a step back and not to push activity after activity onto him. Allow David room enough to be the clichéd slippered old man gazing into the fire if he so choses.

I open the calendar. Empty but for a neurologist's appointment, September's page stares empty—for the moment.

> Feeling guilty leaving for half an hour, but I must get out. People telling me I am being so strong and that he is lucky to have me makes me squirm.. Every morning, resolving to be nice and calm and kind and then some stupid little thing makes me blow my top. Oh I was glad to hear I was not alone on that one   ~Carol

September 2, 2017

44. transition... the Gentle Slide

Seven days have flown since we stepped over the threshold into our home. After six weeks away, with jet-lag gone, bags emptied, our action-packed, timetabled lives loomed impenetrable as a portcullis.

Warm-water Class. Choir. Think Big And Loud therapy. Acupuncture, Parkinson's support group, my breath quickened.

I'd come to hate my life... the forcing of feet into shoes, arms to sleeves, the gobbled meals, and goading it took to make David's appointments on time. Forget mine—ophthalmologist, OBYGN, coffee with a friend—those I squeezed in whatever vacant spot appeared. I'd never learned the art of, "Let the buggers wait. Won't kill them if we're a little late, considering... "

Clocks, timetables, Parkinson's and me — the culprits. My pushing made us miserable. And good times come less often.

"I don't like you shouting," David more frequently rebuked. Unhappy.

By the time we left for the summer at the end of July, my skin waxed pasty, and my spirit shrank depleted. My heart raced. I sometimes dizzied when I stood. And after settling David, often dragged myself into bed unwashed. The sight of me as we stepped from Geneva's Arrivals, had my son and daughter-in-law worrying how much longer I could take this Parkinson's bashing.

David, the Harried and me, the Harrier is how I'd describe us — that is if there is such a word. Truth is, neither of us liked our roles. Even less the people we'd become.

A week in France, and the light returned to David's eyes. Mine too. I'd forgotten the heavenly enjoyment of simply sitting. I traced my gaze along the jagged peaks and glaciers of the Alpine Chaine.

"Ah. More like it. Now I remember... " I sighed kicking off my shoes and settling.

Pure pleasure. Watching life unfold below the farmhouse balcony, the smallest happening became an object to fascinate... Monsieur Charles hoeing weeds from the furrows of his bean patch; Blackie, the family cat mouse-spotting in the meadow grass; a honeybee, feet clubbed with yellow pollen dipping his proboscis into a clover flower. Nature, self, in-tune, connected.

"That's what we should do, David," I spoke, excitement rising. "Bring some space-gazing home."

"Good timing," we laughed, "... to be in the air headed home just as the solar eclipse is happening. By the time we land the sun will have reappeared fresh and newly washed by the moon."

I saw the astrological event as a symbol of our new beginning.

We chatted more. Discussed a gradual honing back. Ridding ourselves of obligations. David's, my, peace of mind was the more important after all.

"We just must slow down," we both decided. "Try and keep our relaxed on-holiday mood going."

Clocks and timetables would rule us no more.

In some Personal Growth-type book I once read, the message I took from it said something along the lines of, "Before anything new can come into your life it's essential to step into a vacuum."

Between genres at the time, and wanting to change the direction of my art from cutting steel to a different medium and style, I sat on my hands. Hardest thing I've ever done... doing nothing. Took me over a year of waiting, waiting... Finally a bag of clay and three-dimensional sculptures formed, and I was off and running.

"I really don't want to take the swim class anymore," David declared last Tuesday.

I stared at his packed sports bag readied for the next day's class. Recalled the pang of regret the day I gave away my tennis raquet. Stammered something about was he sure... was this the right thing to do... what to tell the aide assigned to help.

We'd sort of talked of giving up... but... I was unprepared for the hollow feeling his determination caused me. The rising feeling of wild panic I felt as the scheduled Wednesday/Monday swimming slots erased.

My mind scrambled objections. But, but... Exercise keeps Parkinson's sufferers from decline. Every expert swears the same: To prolong mobility, keep active. David couldn't just sit in his chair and do nothing could he? Or could he? I caught myself.

Whose life was it after all? Could it be my pushing him to fill his day was holding him in a kind of limbo-hell when extended quiet was what he craved. Space to Be. Space to listen. And space to vision and turn within?

How else to prepare for the end journey ahead? Dare I break taboo... voice the words: Dying. Death I see tip-toeing across his mind.

With a start I realized it was me, not David, who was holding on to life. His. And by my keeping him active was unconsciously doing everything I could to keep him with me a while longer.

"Don't leave me," my soul cried, while my mind shook me to face the truth: David's earth-time was creeping closer to its end.

David was getting ready. And I must allow him room to gently fade and go.

Since our calendar has emptied, we've chatted more, been sweeter, more tender even, to one another.

"If there is a heaven, it has a space reserved for you with a handicapped placard," David hugged me to him laughing at his own joke.

That night I dreamed David... *a giant techni-colored Hornbill replendent in a yellow hard hat, with wings so long the tips met beneath his belly as he flapped to keep aloft. Hovering to feed me, he poked a berry as red as his eye through the tree hollow in which I'd encased myself.*

I am so honored to have been the Delta Air Hostess that was a part of your recent journey. Your story has been such an inspiration to me and my family. I shared your blog with my mom who is the caretaker for my dad and she wept as your words became her words.. Prayers for you and your husband as you live one minute at a time with this horrible disease. ~CB.

Thank you for all the understanding and kindness you showed us on the long flight from Europe. I wonder how many of us there are, who like your mother, at 83, should be enjoying a little TLC of our own, but instead are forced to bear the physical and emotionaly exhausting burden of caregiving alone? Her response to my words is I suppose the reason for my writing this blog...to voice those things we caregivers feel but rarely say. ~Liz

45. to truly exist...

… to truly exist… I reread the quote. It keeps me going. Who would have guessed how difficult I would find it.

The opposite of my Father's favorite dictum, *Do as I say not as I do*, I've taken the first tentative steps along a new and slower track. Put my slow-down into action — well, non-action. Quite scary, actually — turning the clock-face to the wall, erasing those two swimming classes from the calendar, and pulling on the breaks whenever I catch myself running. And surprise, surprise, the world has not tipped off its axis, and no hole in the earth opened to swallow me.

First to go. Swimming Class. Why did I resist canceling the class when in truth I hate swimming pools. The way their waters crinkle my fingers tips. Hate the cold-tiled walk to and from crowded changing rooms and their weak-streamed showers. Cost me half a day. Backwards forwards three-quarters of an hour each way.

If duty and being good for the both of us was not reason enough to hold me, why was I so bothered by freeing up those two half days? Took some contemplation, but I think specific classes and appointments act as a kind of anchor for me, markers if you will, to get me through the never ending blur of caregiving.

No problem for David. He is happy to sit for hours with his eyes shut not moving a muscle. TV either on or off makes not much difference to him.

No surprise he was awarded the Buddha prize at the end of our ten-day white-water trip down the Grand Canyon.

"You go. I'll stay here." He turned down most side trips preferring instead to still cross-legged at the river's edge and contemplate.

Not me. Awarded the most improved camper, my time was spent in terror skirting death by whirlpool, ice-water rapid, and fall from knife-edge precipices. The guide even had us abseil down a cliff face we'd climbed by rope. Uggh. I still quake remembering. Never said my prayers so often.

David is still that calm man from all those years ago.

"Better do it. Call to cancel," I checked the swim aide's number and dialed, finding it strangely stressful telling him he was no longer needed.

"That doesn't sound like David," the young man argued. "He loves swimming."

Clearly, he believed the choice was mine not David's, and I found myself inventing excuses in explanation.

"Are you telling me David is getting ready to die?" He countered bluntly when I explained David wanted to slow down.

"Err, err, um... " I parried trying to unscramble a tangle of unformed and very private thoughts and feelings.

"In a way." I heard the protective seal around my heart crack.

I returned the telephone receiver to its cradle. Sat silent a moment fearful, as if by admitting such a thought aloud, I was inviting death to happen.

"Talk about blunt," I exclaimed brushing away the aide's crass questioning.

David and I had talked of the future. Of course we had. But what we discussed was nobody's business but David's and mine. Private.

David looked up and announced he was ready for more coffee.

"Don't worry. I'm too physically fit to pop off just yet," he comforted.

His pink cheeks and strength confirmed the truth of what he said. Yet... yet... David's spirit wavered.

Since returning from France, both his caregiver and I, have noticed a new vagueness, a sort of disconnect to what is going on around him.

"What are we doing here?" He might ask.

And then there is his obsessive searching for objects he's not touched for months... his car keys are lost, a turquoise ring, bed-side flashlight, or a slip of paper with a scrawled phone number.

Naming *whatssisname*, no problem, David spits the name right out. His mind so clear and focused one moment, next second David confounds me with the off beat ramblings of his mind.

"*Goodbyeee. Goodbyeee. I wish you all a last goodbye,*" he sing-songed over lunch last Thursday.

"*We'll meet again.*

Don't know where don't know when,

But I know we'll meet again some sunny day."

We sang Vera Lynne's war-time lyrics together.

"Where on earth did that come from? Something you practiced at choir?" I asked.

"Just felt like it," he answered, sheepish. "Came in through the window."

Parkinson's held him trapped. One foot in hell. The other cinched to life. To me.

Cancel. Keep. Change. I spoke aloud my mental lists to David.

Cancel classes.
Strict time-keeping.
Downsizing

Eliminate stress.
Keep calm.

The *to-do* and *not–to-do* lists grew.

Swimming…gone. I flipped through September, October, November's calendar. Circled the movement disorder specialist's appointment in Arizona.

"That could go. Are you okay with transferring care to your Albuquerque neurologist?"

Though the winter break would be fun, David no longer needed the stress of more tests, more travel. I remembered the nine-hour drive, the nightmarish effort to pack David's rigid body into the car at dawn. No, those horrors we could do without.

We crossed off October's Parkinson's conference. Crossed off a friend's visit.

"We have too much going on right now," David decided.

Instead of push-pulling ourselves to be on time for last week's appointment, I called the PT's office and announced, yes announced, we were running late.

"We'll be there when we get there," I countered when she rattled papers over the phone. "These forms need to be filled before you can be seen."

"There's plenty of time. I'm speedy." I stood my ground. Scored a point. Proud of myself.

Scored another…

Hard for a pack-rat, I winced as I cleared the dark oriental cushions from the banco immediately brightening the living room. Encouraged by the effect I scanned the walls, the mantle piece and coffee table.

"Next to go… pictures, knick-knacks, sculpture… at least some. Oh to be Zen."

I emptied my maybe-wear-them-one-day clothes into a black bag and hid them from myself before regret snatched them back. I swept David's unworn underpants and socks into a bundle for the men's homeless shelter. I've yet to tackle my grocery cupboard.

I'm usually awake and dressed an hour or so before David stirs.

We've always breakfasted together however hungry or bad-tempered waiting for him often makes me, even those mornings his eyes stay shut and I have drag him from bed to bathroom and lead him to his chair. By then starving and frustrated the ritual begins: One forkful of fruit thrust at him. I snap my jaws for the next. One bite of buttered toast and marmalade for him. One bite for me. Force a sip of coffee between his partially closed lips. I gulp down three.

By the time breakfast finishes my good resolutions to be calm are scraped into the trashcan with his leftover crusts and crumbs. I battled my conscience before breaking my it's-only-polite-to-wait rule and allowing David to sleep in until I've finished my breakfast.

These days alone with the first light of day, I nurse my bowl of fruit, marmalade-laden toast, and mug of coffee wondering why eating in turn hadn't occurred to me before. When David wakes, replenished and calm, I have a second with him.

Two microchips embedded in my psyche drove me as I was growing up. One insisted *idle hands make mischief,* sitting down before the sun beds himself feels too sinful to enjoy. I do take a twenty-minuter — a catnap after lunch most afternoons. "Like Winston Churchill," I excuse myself.

Reinstating my daily meditation, I open book to the day's contemplation.

> *YOUR DHARMA IS TO TRULY EXIST BECAUSE THIS*
> *IS THE LIFE YOU'VE BEEN GIVEN BY GOD.*

Hmmm, i sigh.

46. ...and the world laughs with you...

Goes the saying, but I had no laughs to laugh.

Not moving, not speaking. David leaned back in his favorite chair, his eyes closed. I looked over. I was alone. It was Sunday. Saturday had passed the same. The weekend stretched long.

Isolated in the living room beyond reach of David's world, my mind flipped back to my arrival at the Country Holiday Home for Children, and the feeling of abandonment as we stood rigid, uncomprehending on its doorstep, the two of us, my baby brother and me. Five bewildering years, the paying orphanage was home.

"My mummy's been stolen by a wicked man." I'd say gravely struggling to explain her rejection.

I pushed her face below my consciousness. Drowned her.

Made her dead.

I stared at David's form.

Kidnapped by the Parkinson's thief, only his breathing showed he was still living. It mattered not whether I left the room or stayed. I stood a moment by the door. Then walked into the kitchen.

Suddenly I ached for the mother I'd never had. And for my guardian, Auntie Pat, wishing her back alive to love me. I missed the cadence of her voice, the deep sharings of our girl-talk. I missed her scented aura of Blue Grass *eau de toilette* when she pulled me close.

Of course it was David's love I really sought. His voice I strained to hear. His arms I yearned to wrap about me. But like my father, mother and my Auntie Pat, David, was no longer with me.

At the children's home I wove a safe house high in the broad arms of my beech tree. There I'd climb above the world to a secret place where not a soul could harm me. And leaning against its silken bark pretend the feel of my ayah's sari.

Alone with David last weekend, I had no such refuge. I went outdoors, pruning shears in hand. Fiercely amputated the new growth from the spreading quince tree outside the kitchen window.

Mostly, we have no social gatherings lined up. This weekend we had three.

Saturday, the sitter arrived to be with David, freeing me to attend the village community breakfast. Thought it good to re-connect after nearly two months away. Wrong, wrong, wrong. Hot from the bowels of my morning's caregiving chores, the plunge into a sea of pleasantries and chatter silenced me. The art of banter forgotten, no bright, light words came to mind.

I envied people their easy conversation. Their normal lives. Unable to bear my unease, I munched my green chile burrito and fled.

Later, in the afternoon a friend turned sixty. Her tea party was to be a surprise. David's sitter was nowhere to be seen.

"If I don't leave now I'll spoil the fun," I checked he was safe and sitting down, the TV playing. "I'll have to go, David. The sitter should be here soon."

I made it in time, and crouched in the bushes with the other waiting guests. *SURPRISE*, we cried sweeping the birthday-girl indoors.

With half my mind home with David imagining him sprawled helpless on the floor, I circled the room dropping a few hello-how-are-yous, sipped a glass of tap water, eyed the pristine candles, the uncut cake, the unopened wine bottle, called someone I know really well by somebody else's name, and labored to make conversation.

"Happy birthday. Have to fly." I fled to the car and escaped home.

Next day more of the same. Another friend's birthday. Her seventieth. I arrived late assuming the party a buffet. Not so. Two tables set in her shade-dappled orchard. Eleven upturned faces greeted. Eleven half-finished plates. Eleven poets' voices murmured. Lunch was a sit-down affair. I slipped into the vacant chair and turned to my lovely neighbor hoping to blend in. One on one, she made it easy. An hour passed.

"I must get back to David," the cake cut, and every crumb devoured, I stood, desperate to leave.

I'd like to have stayed. Heard their poems declaimed. To have dreamed with them. But those days of pleasure and leisure were no longer mine to have.

I'm not sure what triggered Sunday's feeling of desolation, all I knew was I felt infinitely sad and utterly alone.

David resurrected, sensed my sadness. "What's going on? Are you upset," he asked, concerned.

That did it. A wail escaped, and I fell into his arms spilling my grief.

"I don't fit in," I sobbed. "I've forgotten how to socialize."

"There, there," he soothed.

As good rains wash clean pollution haze from the desert landscape, so too my tears cleanse me.

More than a little shamed by my outburst of self-pity, I fixed tea, and laid out David's favorite shortbread on a plate.

47. heaven is when you think it is

I can't believe it's working… our invisible transition to live a slower pace. With less must-dos, these past days unfurl as open as a month of Sundays.

Getting up a little later no longer feels I'm committing some hell-fire sin as I was brought up to believe. About time, I'd say after all my years of heart-pounding scurry-hurry from one appointment to the next.

David sleeps in nowadays. What's more, I let him, welcoming the block of *my time* his sleep-in gives me. Take this morning.

My dreams still vivid, and bedroom windows two rectangles of featureless black, I slipped to the kitchen to treat myself to a cup of tea in bed. Propped half sitting, I sunk back against the softness of the plumped bed pillows, blankets pulled to my chin, and waited for day to nudge the night from her path, and reveal the hogback's rocky outline against the sky bordering our property.

For a cherished hour, snuggling down I think over how I'll spend the coming day.

… my mind meanders, but mostly all I want is to sink into the quiet. Feel it. See it. Hear it. Remember who resides inside me.

During my six-week stay at the ashram in Maharashtra State, India, over twenty years ago, my assignment was to rise at two thirty in the morning and help prepare the massive ashram's open-sided meditation hall in time for the first program. From necessity I learned to wind and pleat my sari by feel, grab my woolen shawl, and tip-toe from the dorm guided by a thin beam of my pocket flashlight.

Sounds like a regime from hell, but to me I had stepped into heaven... the magical walk alone in the dark through heady jasmine scented gardens, the soft lights of the hall, the hours of silence working beside my fellow *sevites* until the musicians arrived, and candles flickered to life as the hall opened.

Just before first light, and the sky still dark, each morning I noticed a momentary gust of wind blew from the East heralding the dawn. At first I thought my imagination was playing tricks, but the cold blast blew again the next, and every day.

I wonder if the strange phenomenon occurs in every part of the world or is noticeable only in a warm climate? Or was it noticeable only because I, like Thoreau, took a step back from the world to consciously observe nature's play happening all around me? Whatever the reason, the breath of pre-dawn taught me a great lesson in awareness. In being fully present.

I liked the person I was then: C-A-L-M, uncomplaining, observant, yet detached. If that person still lives, I need her now to help me through these last years, months, weeks, or days of caregiving as I feel my David winding down.

Today, in glorious silence, I'm tapping the computer undisturbed. Ate a plate of homegrown tomatoes, basil from the garden, and mozzarella breakfast while smiling at the antics of the finches in the birdbath outside the window.

Right now the clock reads nine-thirty. I go to check David's still breathing. Note the faint rise and fall of his chest, the sunlight and peaceful glow of his face. I leave him be, and return to my desk. Next I know, a glance at the clock catapults me to my feet.

"Wakey, wakey David," I run to rouse him. "Can you believe the time?"

Reminding myself to keep my calm going, I swing his legs over the side of the bed, guide his hand to the bed rail and help him sit, help him dress and to the toilet, then pop pills and two partials into his mouth without even a shiver, and walking backwards lead him to his chair for a second breakfast. Phew. Made it without feeling ruffled. I pour two cups of coffee. Join him.

"Yup. Nothing on the books today, David. Anything special you'd like to do?" I query, wondering how long we can keep the calendar commitment-free.

How long before we scream from boredom? So far doing much of nothing feels just fine, and today and all this week, the life we've been dealt, in fact seems incredibly halfway good.

Could I actually be enjoying myself?

"How do you feel after such a fifteen hour-long sleep?"

"Great. My body is telling me something," David commented at brunch spooning mouthfuls of black bean stew.

Too late for breakfast, in time for early lunch, he woke a few minutes before midday.

"What is your body saying?" I asked, understanding full well his body's message.

He looked up, and not saying a word continued eating.

What strikes me is how deeply moving the kindness of strangers can be. and how that touches the most vulnerable place in us.. ~JT

September 30, 2017

48. Silence is Golden

"There's always that nice Home Help Agency we interviewed if we can't manage, David," I assured him bravely. "We'll hole up like bees in a hive, and cope fine, just you see."

And with that said, I made a massive grocery run to keep us in food for the two weeks ahead, warned friends we were temporarily out of action, and crossed off a couple of commitments from our schedule.

Friday. Still nothing came to mind for this week's blog. I mean nada, zilch. My mind drew a complete and utter blank.

I scowled at the computer screen. Homebound I had done nothing special, no miracles had occurred, not even scored one Quick-pick number for Saturday's Power Ball, and no disaster had struck us unlike poor Puerto Rico, so what the devil was there to blog?

Would this be the week I failed to honor my commitment to write a weekly blog for one full year. I lay in bed worrying.

What, nothing to report? Was I nuts…? I jumped from bed as events from the past week rolled like an old Pathé newsreel.

Vertigo. Ah yes, I suffered a debilitating attack. How had I wiped such a recent and devastating event from memory? Forgetting exactly what I ate yesterday for breakfast is one thing, but this… ?

Saturday afternoon. My last week's blog posted, and with nothing looming but a cup of tea, I filled the kettle.

"Hey David, how about a drive to town and see that new film, "Viceroy," the one about Partition?" I called out from the kitchen.

But as I poured, the room began to spin. I clawed my way to bed.

"Uhhh. I'm so dizzy," I groaned. "I don't think I can drive."

The vertigo stayed. I felt I might throw up. When I needed the bathroom, I inched my way, eyes shut, with David leading me by my hands. My yoga pin-holed glasses helped some, but how to get David undressed and prepared for bed? I couldn't lift my head and began to cry — just a little.

"Who to call? Who could help us? With our tenant/helper away on personal business, and the Home Help Agency closed, I felt utterly alone. It was Saturday evening. Raining torrents. We couldn't call on just anyone to do anything as intimate as getting David bed-ready.

"Ah, what about our good friend, the girl you sponsored for US citizenship?" I suggested. "Being a fire fighter, she might have some EMT training so won't likely be bothered by your nakedness."

Like an angel she appeared through the slanting rain, took over, put both David and me to bed.

Next day the walls of the room rooted in place. I lay on the living room couch, yoga glasses pushed tight to my nose not daring to move.

Day three, the world stabilized to almost normal and I settled back to the role of David's sole and full-on caregiver.

Weird, but our being glued together day in day out has been surprisingly okay. Perhaps I'm finally maturing to an elderly matron content to sit broody as a hen on a mass of eggs not knowing which eggs will hatch.

Among the addled I include my plan to take a stall at the annual local flea market and get rid of STUFF. When David's sitter unexpectedly cried off forcing me to cancel, there was nothing for it but toss that plan from my basket.

For a few days I ran a madcap fantasy of dragging David with me, and propping him up on the front seat of the car while I hawked my wares. Then reality struck, and though I'd looked forward to the event for a month or more, calm-new-me gave in with barely a grumble.

"Well at least not going forced me to sort out the shed," I muttered after a few explosive curses.

I can't say a pleasure, but in this mode of slow-down I haven't really minded my caregiving's full-on, repetitive duties it takes to get David through the day.

For every little action we able-bodied so casually take for granted David needs my help. Some days, more. Some, less. But whatever, I'm on constant call... to bed, to bathroom to sit to stand, table to chair, chair to toilet, pants up, pants down, teeth in, teeth out, cup to mouth, cup to table... on and on, I can even shave him, and trim his nails.

Here's an example of the steps it takes to help David sit.

No, David, remember what the 'physio' showed you... come on take one more step... keep going... keep going... that's it... right up to the chair and position yourself directly in front before you sit... hold the armrest... no with your other hand, I stretch his arm so his fingers touch... *that's right... now turn... turn... turn once more...* , I pant physically guiding him to rotate.... *right, now back up till the backs of your legs touch... now reach back to the other armrest... now you can lower yourself... slow... control remember... hurrah you made it, now you can sit.*

Caregiver-me goes through similar motions on auto-pilot. Wife-me rubs his bald head, strokes his hand and comforts,

"It must be awful for you, darling. Being so helpless. It's a hell of a disease."

At the close of week one, our neighbor came over for a good old natter over an evening glass of wine and cheese nibbles. After our self-imposed isolation I looked forward to her company. David astounded both of us with his spot-on comments and political insights. Breaking off mid sentence, he looked wistful for a moment, then said,

"I feel foolish not being able to join in your conversation as much and as spontaneously as I'd like."

The neighbor and I both fell silent, feeling bad… feeling sad.

"It's our fault," we both rejoined at once "… for gabbling on and cutting across you before you have space to form your words."

But, as I said earlier, *life ain't 'alf bad* when we are closeted together beyond life's cruel knocks with time to share our thoughts. Both spoken and silent.

One afternoon last week, sitting on the bench out front cloud watching, we had the thought that perhaps if we listened intently, the white and grey streaking the sky would spill an unspoken message… Something about creation and destruction, maybe? … the form and the formless?… impermanence? Our minds ran.

What would John Francis hear or see, we wondered — the activist who walked rather than ride any gas-driven vehicle, and spoke not a single word for seventeen years? Imagine taking a vow of silence for such a chunk of time. Having watched a YouTube video of his Ted-talk recently, nether of us can get his message of silence from our minds.

Back to plans that go awry, to hurts I cannot protect David from — the phone never rang, and the much anticipated visit of his daughter never happened. Seeing him hunched so crestfallen, I quickly arranged a two-night escape to visit his cousin at his cabin in Colorado.

"He's been begging us to visit before winter sets in," I interrupted David's reverie.

The sun was still up and tangerine when we pulled into his driveway, and the river wildly brown and running. Warm enough to sit on the deck, we settled with his cousin and two dogs to watch a Swanson's Hawk hover, then plunge to the river. Sending up a plume of spray he soared skyward and without missing a beat, circled away over the hay fields apparently unfazed by his failure to score dinner.

A John Francis silent lesson in determination and acceptance, I mused.

That night thunder roared and lightening split apart the sky releasing cascades of torrential rain lasting the entire day and all next night. Our planned soak in Pagosa's thermal springs would have to give way to an indoor day.

David asked for his chair to be pulled up close to the picture window. "I want to watch the rain," he smiled, and he did, the whole beautiful, silent day.

I curled on the settee and read a friend's book from cover to cover. Something I've not done for years — if ever.

We returned home happy and replenished.

No sign of our tenant, but an email from David's daughter awaited.

"She wants to see you. She's coming in November," I called.

… And I thought I had nothing to blog about this week…

How did this happen? a fantastic life up until just a few years ago. it is only in the last two years that things have become more challenging. For this I am grateful and so is he. ~JT

49. nice Girl turns not so nice

I have never thrown a plate or glass to date, but as I emptied the dishwasher oooo how I wanted to hurl the whole damn pile of plates crashing to the tiled floor.

"I've had it. Absolutely had it with all you lousy flakes." I yelled startling David.

God I felt mad. Mad at everything and everybody.

Teeth snapping, and mouth twisted like a snake, my rage caught me by surprise. Shocked, I paused standing for a second, then, calmer stacked the clean plates neatly in the cupboard.

From where had such a temper erupted? At whom was it directed? Or what? Perhaps a result of too long behaving *nice*, as Americans so ungrammatically are fond of saying?

I thought back through my day — how I tip-toed through the tulips so to speak — my careful dance around this friend's fads and foibles, the solar-man's timetable, the capricious non-appearance of the guy who promised to help clean up our yard before the village Studio Tour. The therapist's delicate feelings.

"Oh, hi. I'm a little worn out today, I'll have to cancel."

"The accountant is out of the office so your claim is on hold."

And, "I do better traveling with a friend. How are you fixed next month?" His out-of-state beloved, I won't name but you-can-guess-who asks to re-schedule.

"What about David's feelings for a change, you selfish cow? And a consideration for my needs would be nice?" I want to shake her, and all those *La-las* unable to stick to their commitments. "Ever wonder how I'm managing alone?"

My eyes rove the littered papers covering dirty plates and cutlery on the dining room table, the open jar of marmalade still there since breakfast, the dregs of coffee cold in their mugs, the crumbs of toast...

Too much to deal with. I just can't cope. I force David's shoes over the heel of his stockinged feet, get him standing and push-pull him towards his T.V. chair.

"Come, David. One. Two. Left. Right. Move those feet." I snarl my frustration onto my poor long-suffering David.

Of course, like all good girls I bite my tongue. Don't yell what I'd really like to spit down the phone.

From inside a head of steam headed up my throat makes it hard for me to breathe. With one mighty poof... the expletives exploding from my mouth shock even me.

Like the worst of all thunderstorms, my anger subsided and thankfully so too, my nasty mood blew over.

When self-pity overwhelms me, I try thinking how it must be for David. Of his impotent frustration. How the devil does he keep his cool? I, at least, have choice.

I imagine the highborn Chinese women born at the time when society deemed bound feet desirable — feet so mutilated as young girls, they were never able to run and walk after their mothers cracked and snapped broken their bones. I've never forgotten the account of a five year-olds' wails of agony and rage in a book called The Fan.

When I think of my own childhood in Devonshire, how I'd have felt deprived of my freedom to jump and run, I run dry of complaints.

Peace settles. David and I stroll the driveway. Offer a windfall apple to the neighbor's horse.

＊　　＊　　＊

I remember her, me the child
index finger horns pointy on her head a billy-goat
unafraid inside a druid's sheep-cropped stone
circle bounds the moor crushing purple heather
feels wind's wild comb un-tangle her brown hair
balanced on one leg atop Kestor's granite outcrop
'I'm the King of the Castle' she sings
to no one for no reason but to feel song's
quiver strike not a bull's eye but a raven's

＊　　＊　　＊

Wednesday, October 4th, catastrophe struck.

Late evening we watched the clouds loom black. The heaven's fired near golf-ball-sized ice bullets at our skylights breaking four. Rain torrents slid the three hillsides behind our house and forced its way under the doors, between the outside wall and ground… any way it could. Crack-crash, the sky lit up and plunged David and me into the dark.

The well pit filled with flood water and blew the well pump. I paddled through two inches across our studio-den to check the electric breakers.

Our tenant, unable to open the door against the eighteen-inch wall banked against it, climbed through the window and paddled to help us stem and mop the impossible.

One bedroom and half the living room escaped. David sat marooned in a solitary chair, feet on a stool above a carpet-less floor for two full days confused and quiet.

Caregiving? This caregiver's job was to keep him calm, to keep him fed and cared for him on schedule while all around him reigned chaos. Our kind cleaner's husband appeared with a helper and busied filling sandbags, digging the existing channels ever deeper and rebuilding the collapsed berms. Meanwhile our cleaner and a young couple helped swab and mop the mud.

When Wednesday's storm struck, all our petty hurts and troubles vanished as nothing. Not the method I'd have chosen to rid oneself of anger, but it surely worked.

Yes. caregiving is hard particularly on too little sleep, but all we can do is to have good intentions to do the best we can. Every day I swear I'll be patient and help in a gentle way. Every day something trips me up turning me momentarily into a person I don't want to be. We too have become isolated so I sympathize. ~KJ

50. the aftermath

In the wake of Wednesday's flood, the next morning revealed a tideline not only in our house but the shed where we stored paintings but had no room to display on our already crowed walls…

The paintings we planned for ten past years to sell one day but never quite got around to doing, now stood sad and soggy in the residue of mud, too be-spoiled to market.

I can't tell you how many times we swore to make a list and contact the galleries representing the artists. Even got as far as photographing and measuring them before running out of steam and restacking them.

"Hey ho… that's one way to downsize," we comforted ourselves ruefully smashing the cracked picture glass and dismantling the frames to decide what if any of the art was salvageable.

The lesson to not put off till tomorrow what you can do today stung. The mental list of the must dos loomed so drear and long, I wondered if we'd live long enough to complete it.

"Won't bother me when I'm dead. Let other people deal with things," my mother's eyes would glint as she raised her glass with a *Cheers*. Her attitude had shocked me then. Hmm. I understood better now.

Time has been on my mind a lot of late… the sin of wasting something as precious as time with David.

I want us to spend not only quality time together, but share the mundane daily minutiae of our lives.

But what is a waste of time I question? I worry I have I sinned by wasting time and neglecting poor David these post-flood days, though I know I really had no choice while I mopped and swept to get the house and studio ready in time for our annual village Studio Tour.

Yup. On top of the flood, the Studio Tour—a weekend when hundreds of strangers flock to look at, and finger your A-R-T and, if you are lucky, buy.

Treasure the time you have for not even the wealthiest man on earth can buy an extra second, today's entry in my book of contemplation read.

I felt a twinge of guilt... thinking my time would be better spent tending David, rather than fiddle-faddling getting the house in order and displaying my sculpture and books, for two full days chatting up strangers with the hopes of scoring a sale.

More often nowadays I want to stay around David. I worry if we are apart.

Take this week's blog. I haven't had a chance to write these past ten days. And here I am ignoring him after all this time of being too busy to do more than fly past with an, *everything okay darling?*

So please excuse this short epistle... I hear his whistle calling.

"Goddamn it, David. Give me five more minutes to finish up."

OOOps, didn't I say time cannot be bought, much less given?

51. think Loud and biG

Over hearing the title of the Parkinson's exercise program THINK LOUD AND BIG, my ears pricked alert.

Living outside the box and thinking big is something I've been trying to do all my life — more recently, how to make bearable the cruelties of Parkinson's disease.

Hadn't I done this all before? Was this a replay so I could get it right this time? Wife to carergiver, mother to therapist. Can't my relationships ever be normal?

Way back, a mother for the first time, when my baby's Profoundly Deaf diagnosis felled me to my knees, if it hadn't been for the innovative ideas of an Australian therapist, my son would never have acquired the fluent lip-reading and verbal skills that enable him to move between the hearing and deaf worlds as he choose. Deaf education was limited then to conventional signing methods of communication.

✳   ✳   ✳

Without expecting a magic cure, when David's head shaking turned to a *page-jiggling* nightmare fifteen or so year's back, and his voice faded beyond the range of human hearing, we scanned cyberspace for Ayurvedic centers. spread out a world map, decided on India, and made a couple of reservations. Launching into the unknown we signed up for the twenty-eight day's stay in a Kerala Ayurveda nursing home as prescribed. Quite a leap for an allopathic medical doctor, but David gamely committed to comply without question to whatever treatment plans the doctor set for him.

Not to be a pussyfoot, I signed up as well with the hopes of reducing my increasing crippling bouts of diverticulitis and colitis.

Twenty-eight days later, our treatment over, we checked out and headed for the Indian Ocean... David with a strong voice and no head tremor... and me able to eat all the burning spiced and gas-producing pulse foods and nuts denied me for so long.

Agreeing to an alternative Ayurvedic *ghee-in-the-eye* treatment for early cataracts wasn't as easy. After all, he is a medical doctor. The warm ghee stung like the devil but in less time than it took to boil an egg, David saw colors he'd never seen before, and I counted each blade of grass from a hundred yards.

After nine years, cataracts are again slowly drawing their protective veil between our eyes and the UV rays of the New Mexican desert.

I'd be up for returning to India for another bout if it wasn't for David's inability to endure the long hours of travel.

Then there was the off-beat program of seemingly foolish and unrelated to the eye exercises we agreed to practice for half a year, that gave David back such good vision he was able to spot a distant eagle. (see Blog no: 6. A Vision Quest.)

Yup. Life beyond the confines of convention is stimulating to say the least.

We are not ready to turn our backs on new ideas just yet.

*   *   *

"Hey David... Come check this out." The month was May. I beckoned him towards the computer screen.

Our mouths dropped open as we watched the before and after video of a man's struggles to don his jacket — one agonizingly laborious minute before his course of LSVT, twenty seconds after.

"Wow. Imagine you learning to do this."

We goggled together watching a couple of other Think Big YouTube videos.

The premise of their program made total sense. So many of David's movements had shrunk over the years. Letter formation for example. His writing now a tiny scrawl indecipherable from the scratchings of a bird's beak on Aspen bark; the stride of his walk, a shuffle with the lift his feet gone, one arm hangs limp. David lost the ability to switch balance from one to the other leg. When we walk the drive, he often stoops nearly doubled with his face parallel to the ground.

The local LSVT Big Practioner's goals were first to build back David's basic skills to give him better control of his movements before attempting more complicated tasks like getting up and holding a glass simultaneously.

Sitting in on therapy sessions I watched and learned the repetitive tactile and verbal clues David needed to re-pattern his stand-up-sit-down, to straighten his posture, correct his body's left tilt, to switch balance and weight change from leg to leg.

The first time I watched him stride around the gym arms swinging I clapped and almost cried as his hesitant shufflings changed to near-normal strides. Rejuvenated by his success, round and round the therapy gym he circled in victory laps.

The therapist walking backwards held a pair of hiking poles and manually swung David's arms till he could take over on his own. We do the same now on our daily turn up and down the drive.

One. Two. Left. Right.
Swing those arms. Lift those feet.

Miracles in the therapy session are one thing. Quite another when they materialize at home.

Though I've raised the height of the seat, and David still struggles to rise out of his chair, I no longer have to use my last ounce of strength to bodily haul him to his feet. With a light tactile clue and encouraging one, *two three and UP*, he's standing and ready to right his balance before walking himself to the bathroom or wherever.

"Weight over your toes, David. Now bend and lower your butt... " Verbal clues are often enough to get him safely seated, settled.

With no more sessions available this fiscal year, it's up to us to keep up the LSVT practice. In the New Year it may be possible for him to do the intensive course: one-hour-a-day, four-day-a-week, for four weeks, which according to David's therapist, can work amazing results.

LSVT is making our daily lives a whole lot more manageable. My shoulder joints, knees and arm and core muscles are almost smiling at not being stretched to snapping point as much.

I am happier. David delights in his increased mobility.

Best of all, I realized this week we are again doing the no-no things I swore never to do with him ever.

Like go to the cinema, or eat out, the two of us alone. I have the LSVT program to thank for our stress-free outings, for his better mobility and balance. Can it be our lives are improving just as David was ready to slump into apathy.

Yesterday in Albuquerque, David's neurologist stared astounded at his steady footsteps and firm handshake.

"Keep up whatever it is you're doing," she encouraged.

Perhaps next visit David will perform that jacket-putting-on miracle once we learn the steps.

52. You Call this Living?

Well there it is… weekly blog number 52, one full year of caregiving recorded. A good time to take stock and decide the worth of continuing.

This past year David has looped from the depths of depression, paralyzing seizures and immobility, to a man looking and moving so well friends remark on his healthy looks. Yet death has been on our minds… not in a morbid way, but the practical choices we need to make NOW while we are calm in order to avoid hasty choices on what will be the worst day of one of our lives. Yes, his or mine, we have no way of telling.

You see, when we returned home at the end of the summer, David, feeling worn and helpless, sort of decided it was time to fly this worldly realm and he would be unlikely to see Christmas.

"I'm getting ready," he announced recently. "My brother Joe comes and sits on my bed," he paused, seeing something or a person beyond my vision. "He doesn't say much… more often nothing."

When ghosts of the dead come visit the living, I take it as a definite sign.

"Well what things would you still like to do before you go?" I asked as casually as I could, disconnecting my voice and demeanor from the icicles stiffening my spine.

"Think about who you'd like to see… before…

Your daughter of course, and... "

I snuck a glance at David's face. In a household where feelings are not always expressed, his eyes held my gaze. Unwavering.

"I'd like another look at my pre-paid funeral policy," he requested by way of answering.

"You really want me to arrange a cadaver viewing before being in-terred?" My hand shook as I ticked yes to the question. "But why on earth... ?" I stopped myself from asking. After all these were his choices not mine.

"How about a faith-based service? Okay that's a no. So just a few simple words, then?

David liked the idea of a send-off party surrounded by family and friends — a celebration of his life.

Disembodied, we talked of where he'd like his ashes scattered as if we were discussing where best to plant next year's roses or what he'd like for lunch.

I closed my eyes comparing his daily functioning of a year ago at the start of this blog, to his ability today. Recalled the hellish vis-its to public places... the Saturday matinée he froze in the Violet Crown's cinema exit trapping the audience inside... the awkward spills of restaurant food, and being unable to rise from the table... the tell-tale souvenir he left below his chair... on and on.

David's increasing limitations making life no longer pleasurable, it seemed clear — THEN — his body was failing.

I recall the airless hospital room waiting with my son. The intermi-nable night-long vigil while the doctors worked to save him... my mind's eye seeing the word widow fluttering like a neon light on the blink.

Yes, some days the choice I made still bothers me. Was I selfish?

"So did I do the right thing, David, in allowing the doctors to save your life... .induced coma, catheter, and all?"

"Do you wish I'd let you die?"

"No. I'm glad we have this time together. These extra years of life," David reached for my hand.

"Even though you are so disabled?"

I still worry because by now I thought, we both thought for sure David would be dead, and I a widow.

Clearly his body had other ideas. Compared to even six months ago, David is a resurrected man. Uses the toilet even. Impossible to imagine now; for two years before that he wore a catheter, could barely walk on his own, and as for talking... well... three consecutive words rarely passed his lips.

ALL IN ALL, THE WAY HE FUNCTIONS NOW IS A MIRACLE.

How did it happen?

I recognize he has lost weight, tires quickly after any activity or outing, and sleeps a whole lot longer. Eleven hours some nights. His eyes, though they still freeze shut, close less often. I help him stand and sit, lift his legs onto the bed, but thanks to better leg – strength, those tasks cost me way less physically. I have Think Big And Loud to thank for that.

"Hip-hop to the front of the bed," I remind him with a gentle tactile clue. "Walk your feet back under you... now separate your feet... lean forward... push on your hands... now rise up Sir Galahad," I joke, grateful for his renewed effort.

Helping him dress and go to the toilet still costs the same. And reminding him where his toothbrush is, where the car door handle is, and how to lift his cup, the *etceteras and blah-blahs* of daily life still bug me, but overall we are managing sooo much better.

We happily eat out at carefully chosen venues; go alone again to films confident of no mishap to spoil the outing. Ahh... and the conversations the two of us again share make me feel David is back. Impossible to believe, he even chats a little on the phone.

I understand why friends looking from the outside remark amazed at his progress. Yes. I get it. From the outside, overall, David is immeasurably better. But inside?

With a pang, I realized his spirit is slowly withdrawing not only from the world but from me as well. Unconsciously, not wanting to face reality I've spent this year resisting the obvious.

By that I mean his shrinking will to live, and how that has, and IS, affecting my behavior.

Thankfully the rage I described in my first blog has gone except for occasional outbursts, but a crippling sadness has infiltrated my being and stopped my joy. I forget to shower, don't want to talk to people much less see them. And yet... and yet sometimes feel so isolated and alone of an evening when David sits eyes closed withdrawn beside me, I feel already a widow.

"Stay," my darling, I want to whisper. "I want to keep you with me. I'm not ready for you to leave."

Let's face it. Internally I'm a watery wreck.

Yesterday, the autumnal air enticed us outside for a morning stroll. No thought of using his walker as he would have this time last year, with just a pair of hiking poles as support and me close behind ready to catch him, he strode over the rough ground, through the village past my writing friend's cottage, and down the slope into the golden-leafed Bosque.

His gait steady, posture more upright. We stood listening to the *shush-shushing* of the quivering branches of the ancient Cottonwoods, accompanying the creek's gentle gurgling.

"This is where I want my ashes scattered," David squeezed my hand. "Here."

No words. I laid my head on his shoulder.

53. ...and a new beginning

Before I launch into another year of blogging, I decide the time has come to re-sight my intention. Oops, I realized, I don't actually have one... an intention, that is, beyond the vow to speak honestly and to keep going to the bitter end.

"The bitter end?" I brought myself up short. "Now what the hell is that?"

Did *to the bitter end* mean till I run out of things to say, can write no more, or when my caregiving role becomes obsolete with... I fumbled for clarity... when David's life ends and *death doth us part?*

A lifelong commitment, my caregiver's role lasts for as long as David has need of me. So there it is, I have my answer. I'll just keep my "Perfect Servant — nope" caregiver's blog rolling.

As fall glides gently towards year's end, and daylight savings time scares the ghouls and ghosties to slink back into their graves for another full year of sleep, my blog, and ALL SOULS born the first of November, as was my eldest son, rise up to face life anew.

So here we are the two of us, blogger and blogee, an aged crumbling pair, re-shaped and more compassionate hopefully than a year ago, we see one another in a kinder light as valiant warriors soldiering on the best we can.

Re-shaped by stress and the responsibility of caregiving, how could I not be different? So too my best friend and husband, David...

his wings so clipped by Parkinson's disease, how could he not be changed?

I'm not talking of weight or hair loss, but the way the two of us have adapted within our Parkinson's cage. I shouldn't speak for David, but I guess he is more content since we spend more time at home smelling the roses so to speak. I don't remember him ever grumbling or cursing his lot as I do from time to time when depression slays me.

"You can't change some things, darling, life is what it is." David's wisdom floors me. Shuts my grumbling right up.

Thankfully, his pragmatic attitude must have rubbed off a little, for weird to admit, I notice I have settled down to the life I've been dealt. Live more to the quotation I keep on my meditation table.

> *Your dharma is to truly exist, because this is*
> *the life you have received from God.*

"And about time too," I hear you shout back from cyberspace. "How much longer is it going to take to get the message?"

I feel such relief at being able to just get on with whatever task presents itself as it surfaces automatically without resentment. Take those dreaded teeth. It's taken a year but dealing with them no longer bothers me.

"Open darling, and take them out." Sometimes he can. Sometimes not. I wait a second.

As he stands at the basin, my fingers slide inside his mouth and without waiting his teeth head for the running tap.

Never thought I'd hear myself confess I actually prefer being holed up with David flopped in a chair with my shoes and bra flung to the stars. Actually like being a home body.

Yup, I no longer long to be part of the village social whirl. I don't miss it a bit. Don't even feel deprived.

I've always wanted to first glimpse the Taj Mahal holding David's hand as the rising sun strikes its marble domes and sets the turrets afire.

The impossible dream revisits me and I sigh knowing it cannot happen this lifetime. But hey, but how many people can say they've watched dawn break over Haleakalā's black volcanic crater or have ridden the wild white water of the Colorado river as we can?

Can it be that over this year I've clambered from the depths of hell changed but a little stronger?

Without too much thought, I swap out his clothes, mop the spills, pop his teeth in and out without too much of a thought, let outmoded standards slide, and really, truly, I swear, have discovered I'm feeling an overall sense of contentment and gratitude.

Thank you for our lovely home… the sky that's blue… the food on our plates. Thank you for putting up with me. Thank you for being my husband. A childhood prayer comes to mind — the God bless variety.

… and make me a good girl. I remember its ending.

"Now that might take some doing," I laugh ruefully.

I find myself saying almost on a daily basis. I can't believe how selfish-self-centered-unthoughtful so many people I know are and how they abandon us. I know for certain I could never do that, even with my present responsibilities. True to my word I have always been, no matter what. And so dear lady I hope that the coming to a boil actually helped you sizzle and calm down ~Carol

54. Cloud Cuckoo Land

"I'm so much more mellow and calm now compared to a year ago, wouldn't you say?"

I asked leaning forward in my chair with a smile, waiting for my friend to confirm what I had written about myself in last week's blog.

"God, no. Relaxed? Are you kidding? Quite the opposite. I don't agree at all." Her explosive response caught me off guard.

"What? How do you see me, then?" Sitting back, I encouraged her to elaborate knowing I could trust her to speak openly.

"Hyper. Jittery. Some days you're all over the place."She stared at me as though I was nuts.

Whoa, was the new serenity I'd described so smugly the product of wishful thinking? Had my perception of myself as calmer and more content since beginning a year ago been totally delusional?

I didn't defend myself to her, protest, or anything. Part of me uncomfortably recognized she had a point.

By my reckoning David and I had made it through the angry seas and now were gently cruising waters as flat as a millpond.

There's none so blind as those who don't want to see. Same could be said for hearing, I suppose, except in my case I did want to hear.

"Jittery. An utter jitter-bug. You are not offended … ?" Her question trailed unfinished. "I mean how could you not be affected facing such a massively horrendous future with David, and having to deal with all the ghastly things you have to day to day."

"Gracious." I sat back at a loss for words. "Well there's some food for thought."

"It was only when I put my cat down last week," she continued. "... and no longer had to clean up his vomit and messes... he was so sick you see he couldn't use his sand tray... but its only now that I can recognize how I've been dealing with the most horrible stuff for a year."

She was right of course. The only way forward is to ignore the heavy toll caregiving takes on my whole being and psyche when I'm in the thick of it as my friend was with her dying cat. Loving someone does that to us — to me, to my friend. We hate their suffering. One way to minimize it is to just get on with whatever distasteful task needs doing.

I don't want to shame David. Make him feel worse than he already does for putting me through his stuff.

"I desperately wanted my Tootsie's last days to be sweet and beautiful before she was put down. Now she's gone, I just can't believe the ghastly things I had to do to keep her alive and comfortable. Ugh." My friend sat back and made a face. "No more soiled sheets and rugs and scattered kitty-litter my life has returned to normal, I don't know how I did it... and that was just a cat I was caring for."

I listed mentally the unpleasant jobs, which in the normal course of things would slay me... those times I'm forced to wait, socks and shoes in hand my nose to the toilet where he's sitting, uncomfortably folded from the waist while David struggles to remember HOW to lift his feet.

Old me would never have been able to clean him up without my stomach heaving.

New and temporary me — or is new me permanent — just holds my breath and does what needs doing. Doesn't mean I like it. Have to.

And that's that.

"I must be calmer," I argued. "… because in my opinion I've learned to take caregiving in my stride. Well mostly."

Taking stock:

Physically: Stretched and strained to snapping point from doing tasks way beyond the normal capabilities of my aging muscles, is definitely nothing I'd choose if I wasn't forced by David's circumstance.

According to my friends I have more energy than most of them put together. Perhaps my frantic on-the-go and never-sit that jittery side of me was an outlet of my frustration.

Emotionally: Does my constant motion keep me from experiencing feelings I'm unable to deal with if I am to still keep going? My friend says yes. Me? Well I'm thinking about it.

Stretched taut as a violin string I operate in a halfway functional manner, okay, yes I admit it, by keeping distress and outbursts under wraps true British style. Control is how we operate.

Intellectually: I compare myself as a privet hedge, clipped of my natural growth and shaped too neatly for my personality.

Spiritually: Hmm. Not for me to judge.

I think therefore I am… A kind of Descartes — or is it Confucius — conundrum to be sure.

One to contemplate:

If by thinking i feel more mellow, does it mean i am?

241

November 18, 2017

55. itchy feet

"How can you keep going? How do you do it?"

It seems people ask more frequently these days than they ever did before.

It used to be I'd ask the same question of myself. Now I shrug, surprised they don't get it.

There is no alternative.

Too often our Parkinson's Jailor gives a little tug of the thread invisible to anyone but ourselves. I see him sneer reminding us we are in his power.

Knowing struggle only serves to tighten our bonds, David and I accept there is no escape. Like a spider our jailor bides his time, checks his larder is secure. Tweaks his web.

Some days he allows the illusion I have choice. "Go. Go," our Jailor taunts. "You are free to go anytime."

Fooled, I untangle all but the single Parkinson's strand binding my conscience and leave my fellow prisoner for eight whole hours.

David, the man I've sworn to love till my dying day — or his — is deeply sleeping when I depart. I tiptoe past his form fearful of waking him. Fearful of tasks guilt might force me to do if he calls.

Easing myself into a dew-spangled world through the bars of our prison, I stretch and raise my arms towards the rising sun daring myself to run away.

Opening the garage door, it happens. Unfettered by caregiving I become an autonomous adult in a regular world. And hopping into the car am soon on the road winging my way to Albuquerque.

Who cares whether or not the holiday craft and book fair was the right venue to sell my books, I was reveling in the luxury of a whole day off sharing time with my table-mate and friend uninterrupted. No getting David up. No tooth brushing. No struggling to put on his clothes. No caregiving at all.

In an uninhabited stretch of high desert approaching Interstate 25, a lone coyote raises his shaggy head as if to tell me something. A warning? Not waiting to hear, I tramp the accelerator.

"To hell with tricksters, today is mine alone," I sing.

I arrive at the venue by eight a.m. as three air balloons drift over the yellow cottonwoods following the Rio Grande. I wonder how it would feel to fly with them.

"Hello." My friend at the venue was all smiles. "What about a coffee?"

Talk? You bet we did. Laugh? That too. Driving home the Parkinson's thread circling my ankle hung slackened.

"Hello darling," I greet "Only sold nine books, but who cares? I've had a lovely time."

Like Mrs. Average Housewife returning home after a hard day's work, I ask, "And how was your day?"

Freedom tasted good — too good — for me to settle back to life inside the web under house arrest without a struggle. I sniff around for further opportunities of escape, and resolve to bring more of what I wanted into our lives.

My friend was right. I should take little chunks of time for me alone.

I don't suppose the thought of looking for a package deal to the dentist in Mexico would have entered my head but for that remark of hers.

"I wish you could take a little more time to live your own life," my friend looked concerned.

"You're spending more... well all your energy and time on David. What about you?"

"Me?" I looked around.

But like a sailboat on the horizon, I had all but disappeared.

If David were gone, and I alone, could I, would I, find my way back?

Would I really travel to explore the world's wonders of my dreams... retrieve the paintbrushes from their box and fill white canvases with hues I've long forgotten? Would I brush shine into my hair one hundred times a night as I'd been taught at boarding school... or dress fancy just to please myself and because I had the time?

I'd like to think that once... after... David's passing... despite my grief, the ME I am would re-emerge to re-claim those passions of which Parkinson's has robbed me.

"David," I spoke firmly making sure I had his attention as I poured a cup of tea. "I've had an idea... "

That did it. David looked up at me quizzically. A little anxious.

"You know we both need dental work... well, now you don't want to fly any more, how would you feel if I did a quick trip to Mexico? I'm more comfortable going to our regular dentist down in Puerto Vallarta as we've always done. What's more," I checked David's re-action to my spiel, "... I'd get a little break and get my teeth fixed for the price of going to *the damn dollar-thieving dentists* here."

I arranged a sitter for David. Called the dental clinic. Called a woman friend. "Yes, count me in," she assented. I searched for a package deal. Clicked the enter button. She and I leave in two weeks for four glorious days.

The itch I've been scratching abated.

56. thanksgiving... a confession

What a misery guts I've been these past couple of days as the *big American holiday* looms nigh. Yup, that's the one... Thanksgiving.

But what if I'm not thankful? I inquire of myself.

This year the very thought of pumpkin and turkey and all that's orange sets my teeth on edge. As for the *Rudolf carol* belting from the car radio, and forest groves of fake Christmas trees, all tinsel and glitter catching the Indian Summer sun, well, the least said about that...

I flinch, downturn into one of those curmudgeons who hates the premature jolly fun.

Should be thankful, of course. But I'm just not.

Think about it: the endless stretch of road David and I must tread together. No end in sight.

The exit ramp I thought we'd have taken months back by now lies far behind beyond reach. No turning back.

Ahead: thousands of hours' caregiving for me, thousands of hopeless hours' struggle for David.

All we can do is live life out and wait.

WAIT.

Bound as surely as the condemned at Traitors Gate chained to their stakes, like them we wonder how long is left before the Thames River rises to drown them.

So thanks? For what... the bloody Parkinson's chaining him — us — ?

Thanks for the disease's probing fingers picking at the loosening strands on an attempt to rip our tight-bound marriage apart?

Is this what David has worked his doctor's butt off... to spend his hard earned dollars on such an ignominious end after giving so much to his patients?

I can hardly say *life's a peach* and David and I have enjoyed a stupendous year. I mean gratitude to have made it through another twelve months is one thing, but to actually give thanks... So...

NO. Everything is not alright.

NO. I cannot manage.

NO. I'm not strong.

NO. Caregiving is not a choice.

NO. David does not want to end life being manhandled by a fleet of strangers.

NO. Things are worsening. Not getting better.

My body weaker with age cannot survive the physical stress I've been ignoring — hiding from myself.

From my David. From the world.

Somehow we've emerged from last week's black slump. A week when despondency threatened to swallow us. David's emotional strength pulled me through. And mine him.

I'm grateful David is still alive. Of course I am. And for each second left to spend with each other. Grateful I'm still able to care for him at home.

My body, weaker with age, cannot sustain the strain for ever. Just not possible. David, less able too, tries to share the burden, attempts to haul himself to his feet, feed himself the days he can.

We are weary. So very tired.

"I wish I could help you more," he says.

We look at one another.

"Maybe tomorrow will be better," we comfort with hollow words.

Aware this Thanksgiving could be David's very last makes me sad. David too, I suspect. I look over. Notice he's taken to sitting hunched, head and chest almost to his knees.

"Sit up, for God's sake, David," I encourage. "You'll develop pneumonia if you don't. I read somewhere hijacked airplane passengers' lungs fill up with fluid when forced to sit bowed."

I push his shoulders towards the chair back.

Eyes shut, sad, David doesn't — can't — correct his posture.

"Can you hear me?"

He nods as he flops forward for the umpteenth time. I give up.

"I hate this F***ing disease," I sob at breaking point.

"Tell me about it," David's lips part in a wry smile, and reaching for my hands he pulls me onto his lap.

*   *   *

P.S.

Co-joined with good friends around our Thanksgiving table on the day, replete with the best of traditional fare, we raise our champagne glasses, look into one another's eyes and give thanks.

57. turkey bones and magic

Our Thanksgiving dinner long over, my sexy sling-back heeled shoes lie angled on their sides on the mat beside the front door. Scarlet skirt and cream silk exchanged for what I call my slops, the house folds in on itself — silent but for the clatter chink of platters and cutlery as I stack them in the dishwasher.

I thought back to the woman I glimpsed chatting, laughing with her guests, the woman whose eyes brightened with the telling and the listening of lively tales around her table, then slowly faded with the tail lights of her friends' car leaving for their drive home.

Yes, I admitted a little wistfully, that was me I described, the woman I used to be, the woman who used to sing and vibrate the walls with happiness before the three damnable *PAR-KIN-SON'S* rocks embedded themselves with us in our home.

How to keep her? Dispense with the ugly person I've become. At least Thanksgiving has shown me I am still inside there somewhere, and was able to come back.

What could I change in our lives to keep her from disappearing?

I pause, pour off the soup stock from the tangle of boiled turkey bones. Shudder. See myself picked clean of flesh. Bare. Dry. Washed up.

Don't want that person around. Poor David.

My tongue probes my back tooth. Searches for the source of the dull pain.

Excitement surges. A week to go before my Mexican dental trip. The first on my own away from my David for longer than a night since I can remember.

Already I feel the sea ripple up and over my back. Shiver as I rise replenished. My lips salt lick. Miss him beside me watching the sun sprinkle gold water. Run to his arms for a kiss on my return. As we were. Young again… for ever and ever…

Well I can dream can't I?

* * *

MAGIC WORD

the magician holds a card before me
are these the word you wrote he asks
this one
this
I shake my head
spreads a fan of five and twenty images
choose any one you like he leers pushes mine into the pack
but the cards are glued
the magician laughs at my desperate struggle
that night as I prepare for bed
I find my words scrawled on a card
between the cotton folds of my nightie
live now they command

* * *

December 10, 2-17

58. more than $$$

Being a caregiver to my beloved costs no only my energy and sanity, but my pocket as well.

Later today I'm off on my first RNR without David. Nearly canceled when I saw the frightening trail of dollars trickling from our bank account turning my bargain, all-in, three star deal to the cost of a four star stay.

And people with dogs moan the same complaint about the added cost of a dog sitter to their holiday? Try a caregiver on for size.

What with the cost of a replacement caregiver, the extra food and pre-cooking, I wonder if it's worth the trouble just for the sake of four sun-soaked days at the beach?

My heart started pounding. How to get ready in time? What if David chooses to leave... er... *to go...* and I'm not there beside him?

Actually, to my shame I broke down sobbing with the stress of packing, finishing off e-mails, dealing with the futile search of the lost septic permit, scanning documents, making phone calls, writing instructions for the replacement caregiver, making lunch and cleaning up David's accidental mess in the midst of it all.

Micro managing is a bad habit I can't seem to curb. My mind spun.

"I can't go, David," I sobbed through a flood of tears.

"I'm sorry," he indicated the broken glass and sticky mess. "Of course you can. Just go and have a good time. You deserve it, darling."

Immediately I felt like a heel. Worse than the worst of heels.

This blog is short. Please excuse.

I still have things to tick off from my list... put out David's supper... prepare my picnic for the airplane... find ziplock baggies for my toothpaste and shampoo... finish up here and shut down this computer.

I half-wished I wasn't going. Wished I'd stayed in bed. But tomorrow... well... ?

I see myself in capri pants, sand between my toes taking that first delicious sniff of salt and sea.

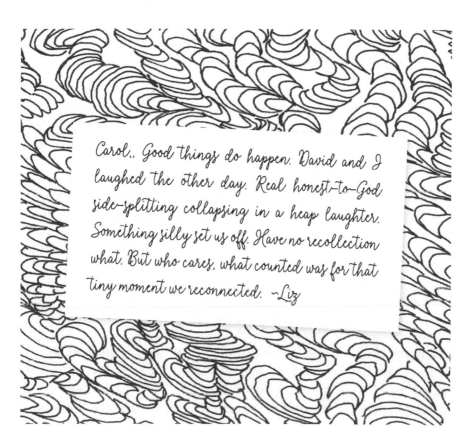

Carol,. Good things do happen. David and I laughed the other day. Real honest-to-God side-splitting collapsing in a heap laughter. Something silly set us off. Have no recollection what. But who cares, what counted was for that tiny moment we reconnected. ~Liz

December 16, 2017

59. Postprandial r & r

Well we both made it.

Five days separation from one another. David home with Caring Caregiver, and me stretched out on the beach, margarita in hand. And, oh by the way, I did have a deep-cleaning and a tooth pulled to justify any residual guilt for treating myself to such a luxury as a mid-winter trip to sea-splashed Mexico.

Foolish me. Before I left, I'd wondered how long it would take me to walk the beach without missing David's footprints beside mine; how long for me to enjoy doing things for myself like watch God's nightly magic show: the sun headed for twilight reddening sea and sky and switching on, one by one, each tiny star.

Guess what? Except for one fleeting moment, it took me two seconds flat. Poof. Unencumbered, I became a whole and independent me.

I can't tell you what a luxury it was to order and eat a complete meal without having to yo-yo up and down spooning alternate mouthfuls between David and me; to step into a taxicab without bundling his limbs off the curb and into place; to dawdle on the water's edge paddling the length of the bay till I tired.

Thinking back to the late afternoon drive to the airport as we headed into the sunset, both figuratively and physically, my travel friend and I shared the concerns we each felt at abandoning our spouse-dependent husbands. Never mind the insistence of friends'

"You deserve a break. You know you do, so just go."

Tossing guilt into the carry-on overhead, my friend and I tucked up our feet and rose into the sky unencumbered as birds.

Soaring, drifting, we skimmed the clouds. Next I knew, a judder woke me. The plane's wheels dropped from its belly and touched down. Foreign soil. Hazy sky. Spanish language. Warm people.

Having left my laptop behind and with no roaming on my cell phone I discovered to my momentary horror I had no email access without being able to confirm my user name or password. I did manage one text to a friend asking her to pass on news of my safe arrival, but that was it. We were both ex communicado.

"Oh, well. Should something go wrong someone would track us down," and with that said my travel friend and I gave up the struggle.

Surprisingly, no withdrawal symptoms descended crippling me. My phoneless phone became a camera capturing images of waving palm trees, startling hibiscus-laden shrubs and the shimmering sea.

Lazy mornings. Glorious indolence I swam the salty sea. Drip dried on the sand. Called for limonada.

Notepad on my lap, the rhythmic in and outing of the tide lured my pencil into the vacuum I've long been seeking but have been unable to encounter at home... the vacuum in which creative thoughts are birthed.

"Ahhh... " words flowed unjumbling.

Eyes closed, reposed on my sunbed, the loose ends of unfinished prequel to my first book, *Poet Under A Soldier's Hat*, jig-sawed into place. A resurgence of energy burned, determining me to find a way to carve a better writing space when I returned home.

After all, I lectured myself, I shouldn't have to leave my own home and head elsewhere in order to find peace and work creatively.

Now if I could plan in some uninterrupted time... Not if, I corrected, it's a must...

Perhaps I could buy two full and consecutive days a month... lock myself away... hand over David's care to Caring Caregiver... I might keep sight of me.

* * *

The second I stepped back home, the happy vibrations between David and Caring Caregiver, hit me. Phew. My five days absence had obviously cruised easily.

My arrival interrupted exercise time. Caring Caregiver, all smiles, showed no signs of stress, and was demonstrating a rotational movement.

David, following her from a chair placed in the middle of the living room, turned to smile at me. Sliding his arm around my waist, he leaned his head against my chest and kept it there as if to make sure I was really back.

"I've been fine. We had a good time," he responded to my quick-fire questioning. "But I'm so happy you're home."

Exchanging news, interspersed with smiles and kisses, we remained glued side by side.

"With you gone, I realize how strongly I love you," his voice cracked as he gazed deep into my eyes.

I squeezed his hands in affirmation, happy to be together once more.

It was true. I was glad to be home. Be back with David. However... I had to confess, while I was away I'd barely given him more than a passing thought, so overjoyed was I to be free.

But as Caring Caregiver headed out the door I felt the heavy cloak of caregiving grip tightly about my shoulders. Squeeze the lightness of being from me. Duties of dressing, feeding, bathing and the deafening slow pace and silence of our lives sent a shiver of dread through me.

A whistle startled me. David's summons? Already? Surely not.

Looking up I saw the yellow eye of a mischievous Grackle, his head tilted mockingly for having caught me out.

That was that… vacation over.

Do your children read your writing? ~N

Not sure. Some do, some don't, some thought it was funny to say "bog off" and ask to be removed from the list. Your question, though gives me pause... makes me wonder if you're thinking its tooooo much information for them to hear? Hmmm.   ~Liz..

Quite the reverse! I was hoping that you weren't hiding it from them. Whilst they may find it an uncomfortable read, I think it is important that the reality of your struggles with PD aren't hidden from them. They will always have a choice of whether or not they want to/are able to read.. ~N

December 23, 2017

60. house arrest

After my break in Mexico, taking up the caregiver's reins hit me hard. The honeymoon of David's and my reunion vanished with the bombshell,

"I'm leaving to be with my family on Tuesday," David's respite caregiver cheerfully announced. "I'll be back in ten days."

I swallowed hard. Counted dates on my fingers. Reality, we wouldn't see her for fifteen whole days.

Panic gripped me. How would I survive being plunged so immediately into full time care?

"How ever shall we manage, David?" I leaned towards him, touched my forehead against his, my hands on his knees. "Fifteen nights, fifteen days house arrest... " I whined. "But looking on the bright side, it means we needn't get dressed from now till Boxing Day."

"Sounds like a vacation," David cheered.

But I was unconvinced. Felt only dread. Strangled by the thought of coping on my own... the thought of the same old, same old... disrupted meals... the constant leaping to my feet to right his glass preventing spills... the repetitive guiding of his spoon towards his mouth... the nights of broken sleep... the heavy lifting of his feet onto the bed... the strain of doing... doing...

A vision of a wild flock of green parrots streaming through David's and my rented *palapa* on their daily flight, flitted from a memory of a Mexican holiday above Playa La Ropa's beach spent over fifteen years ago. I heard again their happy squawkings as they streamed passed. Then imagined the agony of those captured for sale and hung caged in hotel lobbies for tourists' delight. And I, one of them, felt the pain of such a bird.

After my short whiff of freedom, caregiving duties loomed more onerous than ever.

"… and just as I'd vowed to be more calm, and promised myself to better balance time for David, between time for me. Hell and bloody hell." I cursed.

Frowning, scrubbed my well-laid plans for taking uninterrupted stretches of writing time and again relegated my own needs to bottom of the list.

The phone rang.

"Yes?" I barked.

"I'm calling to remind you of tomorrow's appointment with… "

"No way. I can't possibly make it there. I'll have to reschedule," I cut off the receptionist's kindly voice.

Immediately felt guilty. Regretted my nasty temper. Wasn't her fault, poor woman, I felt overwhelmed.

Phone in hand, I eyed David's sightless attempts to find his mug of coffee and pushed the mug against his hands. Followed his fingers' halting creep across the table, his failure to locate the mug's handle. Unable to bear the tragic fumbling a second longer, I tilted the mug towards his lips so he could take a sip.

A surge of hopelessness made me question the point of David's living like this.

Question the nightmare existence of our situation.

The interminable distance remaining ahead.

All at once, I ached to be with my children and grandchildren for the holiday, to be included in their noisy fun — the madcap tearing of wrapping paper, the turn-telling of silly jokes found inside the destroyed Christmas Crackers, or Pulls as Americans call them.

Most of all I yearned for the family that once was mine—my son in England, and one in France, their faces glowing, cheeks reddened from too much good wine at the festive dinner table. I desperately wanted a bite of my daughter-in-law's home grown sprouts, the snap and crackle of crisped pork crackling, and for the warmth and smiles of my three grandchildren.

Yes, I ached, homesick for family with a pain of separation I'd not felt for years.

On the Mexican beach, two weeks back, I'd experienced a little tinge of envy of those families and couples who still had someone to share their lives.

Watching and eavesdropping conversations and interchanges between holidaying couples, forced me to recognize how aberrant our relationship had become with its glowering mood-swings, unnatural silences and stresses.

How quickly I re-adapted to doing for myself and me alone when I left for Mexico, I sighed with unfulfilled longing.

I live alone. Though my David is still with me, in so many ways he's not. Those four days away exposed that sad truth.

My body already hurting from moving him from chair to table, my hand moved to my neck attempting to rub away the pain and ease the tightness of my shoulders.

How long could we endure this hell?

My mind roamed seeking help. Was it time to ask for Hospice Care at home or should we break our vow and move to a Residential Home? My desperation surfed the choices and passed on ashamed. How quickly I'd fallen back into the dysfunctional marriage of David's and my lives. I tell myself to buck up and pull myself together.

Life's a conundrum.

Dread. Yearning. Freedom. Bondage. Contentedness. Misery.

Half of me so happy to have David to share my life, I want us to be together for ever, yet too often half of me dreads such confinement.

Watching David's struggles, and dealing with them and mine, some days I wished him at peace—gone. For his sake as much as mine.

"How can you tolerate life like this?" I ask him sadly. "How can you bear being so helpless?"

"It's not up to me. I have to live out what time I have left the best way I can." He pulled me up short.

Resigned to a choice of one, I turned away.

Maybe, I mused, when David's caregiver gets back, I can find again the person who only last week rode the swell beside six pelicans, and floated in the sea, her face tilted towards the blue expanse of sky.

Hola Carol and thanks for responding and letting me know you too are bothered if not furious when people don't stick to their word. I suppose they have no idea how much we caregivers RELY and count on people actually doing what they say. ~Liz

December 30, 2017

61. happy holiday... oh yeah?

Well of course in the end we did manage to get into the holiday spirit and have a darn good time by throwing a Boxing Day party for close and loving friends. Made up for the eyes-shut-hell and silence of the least Christmassy Day I've ever spent in my life. A day so difficult, the details of which I choose not to recall.

Party Day dawned.

Like Gabriel, an angelic neighbor descended to the rescue. Calmly helped me with the last minute panic that always precedes a party… the unwrapping and setting up of plastic dinner ware, decanting of chutneys, sweetmeats, the chopping of coriander, cucumber, tomato and other condiments to accompany the East Indian curry meal I planned to serve.

Major jobs done, Gabriel roused David from bed, dressed, breakfasted and shaved him.

Corks popped as the first guests tumbled through the door. Bearing smiles and happy greetings their mood brightened the room with light that rivaled the fairy-lit and silver tinseled tree bedecked with glowing chile peppers.

I eyed David engrossed in conversation with another Parkinson sufferer. Connected by the mutual common ground of tremoring they sat close, easy together, perhaps relieved at not having to hide their devastating symptoms. I can only imagine what the two of them shared. No pretense needed, like me when I'm with my Blighty friends. Together for a good old natter over a glug of warming *glühwein* we fall into colloquialisms only understood by us. See what I mean?

Back to Jolly Cheer and Seasonal Spirit, though I say it myself, my Boxing Day Party really was fun. Each friend a kindly Santa Claus, I felt myself believing in the Christmas miracle again just as I had my second, but first ever Christmas I remember in England. I was eight, parentless and only one year off the ship from India.

A CHRISTMAS STORY

Too young to know better, in the midst of pre Christmas fever – pairs of children snipping, cutting gaily-colored paper into strips, another stirring pots of watery flour into a gooey paste, and looping the sticky strips to long paper chains – so engrossed were we with the serious job in hand, a lull fell.

"I am too old to believe in Father Christmas any more." I very clearly and loudly announced.

Didn't stop me though on Christmas Eve from hanging up one of my knee socks on the metal rail at the end of my bed along with all the other children. Or from the excitement of waking to a red balloon tied floating above a bulging sock stuck with a gold Christmas Cracker in the opening; then the trembling exploration of my fingers to the mysterious silver-foil-covered tangerine in the toe, the bundle of crepe paper tied with ribbon – inside a clutch of sugar almonds, hazel nuts and fudge – the discovery of a paper trumpet, a lead pencil, and most precious of all a miniature celluloid ballerina to hang about my neck.

"Father Christmas must have come with his boots off," my friends exclaimed awed, for not one of us had seen him.

I kept my mouth tight shut as by then I wasn't quite so not believing, though not quite believing either.

Way out in the countryside of Devonshire, a county of moors and windswept hills, my younger brother and I shared home with a fluctuating gaggle of between five and seventeen children.

A sort of paying orphanage, Thornworthy, a large, rambling English Country House housed the offspring of those parents whose work took them overseas for years at a time. Abandoned some might say, and not wanting to be hampered, my father handed us into an Auntie Baba's care and sailed for Ethiopia.

Our new mother figure, Auntie Baba ruled with a slipper, the hard backside of her hairbrush, and prayers loving us the best way she knew. Scared as we were of her we took shelter beneath her wings. Belonged.

A bit like the nursery rhyme… There was an old woman who lived in a shoe, and had so many children she didn't know what to do, Auntie Baba lost track, and I turned feral.

Known as the Bad Winter of 1947, snow fell darkening the windows of Thornworthy's ground floor, and sealing the doors with drifts so deep we had to be dug out.

A memory flashed before I could prevent it – me, Mummy, the squeak of our skis tracking the snow, the winter spent in Gulmaarg, Kashmir, high in the Himalayas. Shared laughter.

Isolated four miles from the nearest village, for nearly

two whole months we children were volunteered into collecting bread and groceries by toboggan from the closest drop off point the other side of a steep hill over a mile away.

Tramping and laughing at ourselves, we sank in the deep snow. Together with Jennifer, Jane, Ian and my best friend Norman, I made forays into the winter wonderland to snip great armfuls of blood-red berry-laden prickly holly leaves from what we could see of the buried hedgerows.

Reaching tall as I could stretch I pulled a bough of mistletoe clinging from the hollow oak tree in Home Field. I still recall the white flesh, its squelchy stickiness between my fingers. Winged bows. Leaves of olive-green. Pale as my, and my mother's eyes.

I don't remember Christmas lunch itself, but it was while we were still sitting around the massive dining table still wearing our paper crowns, and having a rare good time and a laugh playing a hand game of Up Jenkins with a silver three-penny bit and a farthing, that I heard them — BELLS.

"SH! SH! Children," Auntie Baba exclaimed cupping an ear with one hand. "LISTEN. Sleigh bells. Can you hear them?"

"Tinkle. Tinkle."

Louder by the second, the unmistakable sound of bells. All of us could and became ever so quiet as with eyes wide as shillings, they were getting closer.

Pushing back our chairs we dashed to the window crowding to peer into the dusk of grey, winter sky. No sign of the sleigh out there.

"He must already be at our chimney," Auntie Baba announced. "Hurry children, let's go into the Smoking Room and see if he's there."

Normally taboo, we children rarely entered the hallowed environs of the Smoking Room, not because of smoking, but because the room was reserved for the staff help.

The maroon velvet curtains were drawn closed leaving just enough light to see. As we pushed and shoved each other to be the first inside, Auntie Baba called out excitedly shushing us.

"SHUSH! SHUSH! I think he's here."

I felt a beetle creeping my neck and my legs started to tremble, for to my terror little pieces of soot began falling into the fireplace, and from inside the chimney breast came the faintest, then stronger and stronger scratch, scratching.

Then, horror.

One black toecap of a boot appeared, then a second followed by two red – trousered legs swinging back and forth, until with a plump Father Christmas dropped into the fireplace pulling down a bulky sack behind him from the chimney.

White beard and eyebrows, the reddest cheeks and nose just like all the pictures I had seen. Father Christmas. He was real. Luckily, there was no fire laid and burning in the grate that day.

All us children had stiffened as the first flakes of soot fell, and backed away fearful not knowing what was scrabbling in our chimney.

Alan, the youngest of us, even screamed.

Without a "HO! HO! HO!" But in a trembly, old man sort of voice, he called,

"Me-rry-Chri-st-mas-chil-dren. Me-rry-Chri-st-mas-to-you-all," he waved.

A little bit less scared by then, we waved shyly back too surprised to speak.

It was then that he asked a question that almost stopped my heart dead.

"Ha-ve-all–the-chi-l-dren–been–g-o-od?"

Auntie Baba turned, gazed at each one of us, one by one, severe and unsmiling.

Recent dreadful deeds came vividly to mind: I'd crawled into the attic and fallen through the ceiling: I'd try to fly, stealing one of Baba's umbrellas and had turned the spokes inside out: Worst of all, I had said out loud that I did not believe in him, in Father Christmas.

I held my breath.

Reaching into his sack, he pulled out a green and red covered package and handed it over to Auntie Baba. Smiling now, checking each label, she called out a name before handing it back to Father Christmas.

"Jennifer!" He repeated, "Merry Christmas!" and beckoned her to come and take her present. "Peter!" it was his turn." Anna!" " Norman!" "Guy!" then my brother Mike and so on and on. The sack became floppier and floppier.

"What about me? Had I been too naughty? Oh please, I promise to be good. I'll be a good girl." I repeated silently over and over again.

Just as I was ready to burst into tears, I heard,

"Is there an Elizabeth here?"

He hadn't forgotten me. I moved shyly to shake his hand and accept my present, the very last package. I don't recall what it was that he brought me, but whatever it was did not matter.

After distributing a mince-pie and a chocolate each, it was time for Father Christmas to leave. Baba escorted him out through back lobby and kitchen to his sleigh.

"It's parked outside the back door," Auntie Baba told us "Watch from the window and wait there until you hear his sleigh bells."

Jingle. Tinkle.

In one mighty swoop and a rush, seventeen faces crowded the window staring up into the black starless sky.

Was that a speck of light I saw? In it Father Christmas shaking the reins of his sleigh? Was that him geeing his reindeer ever higher up and up into the sky? His voice I heard fading with a Ho! Ho! Ho!

❋   ❋   ❋

Happy Holiday.? Oh yeah… this year, with my friends and David around me, how could I not believe in Father Christmas again?

January 6, 2018

62. Goodbye 2017... hail 2018

Final day of the year. Waking, I lie back against my pillow. The house hovers quiet, holding its breath. No bulldozer churning the grey dawn outside my bedroom window for the first time in weeks.

I turn my head staring into the swimming-pool sized hole, the exposed cement cover of the septic tank with its solitary riser, and towering mounds of earth-spill running the sixty feet of trenched leech field.

I sigh. Want all signs of ugliness gone.

Like the frustrations and angry memories of our difficult year, the torn land waits to be backfilled, waits for the earth to cover its scars and allow the healing to begin.

As for us... I close my eyes. Freeze-frame images; me laughing at David's face, his nose wrinkled as he tries to escape the sea lion's fishy kiss. Us: posing a handsome and smiling couple. Healthy. Young.

There's me: chic in a veiled hat, David proud at my side, smart in a suit and flashy tie obviously in love. Happy carefree years. So many good memories rise to the surface.

I study the lone septic riser. Liken its solid, cement structure in my mind to David. To me. Our marriage. The core part of us that withstands. Built firm, brick on brick, rooted straight and tall, like us, survivors of the past's unspeakable sh... t.

Perhaps put off by December's steely frost all the birds must still be sleeping, for I hear no morning birdsong. The stillness is so loud David's purrings travel the monitor across the hallway and drop softly into my room.

I want to stay in this silent heaven forever. Between an end and a new beginning.

Eternity, the Master's say, *lies between two breaths, between the na-no-second of an inhalation and exhalation.*

I roll onto my back and pull the duvet over my head. Focus on the slow rise and falling of my breast. Doze another dreamless hour.

David's bell springs me into action. The last day of 2017 begins.

I'm not sure I want 2018. Dread it if I'm honest. Forget making a resolution for the New Year. I'll be doing well if I can somehow limp through the 365 days.

Hmmm... survive another year of caregiving. Perhaps that's my resolution — to just survive a year that promises to be more difficult than the last with a burden that's likely to increase in weight as David's physical symptoms worsen. His mental capacity too.

More and more often I might as well be speaking an alien tongue for it seems he doesn't understand what the devil I'm saying.

"Pull the door shut," I say, and stare aghast as his hands fumble along the roof of the car, or his fingers over the dashboard.

"If you can't see where the door handle is," I yell in frustration, "then use your goddamn brain. Move your hand up. Up. Below, not above the window."

What shall I do if he looses all comprehension? Or becomes totally immobile?

"But that's not happened," I rein in my wild imaginings. Push away my fear of the trials about to come.

Will this be the year I'm forced to stand alone? Will this be the year Caregiver duties break me? Will David... Will he see another year?

We've talked a great deal these past days. David and me. Life. Death. Heavy stuff. How we'll cruise his remaining lifespan. The future we have left. His mostly. For bar an accident or catastrophic event, let's be honest, I'm more likely to outlive my David.

"I calculate you'll be around two years at the very least. You're so strong," I'd sighed in mid discussion last week.

"Two weeks, more likely," David countered. Startled me with his conviction. I shuddered at the memory of the infinite sadness clouding the room. How we looked at one another. Smiled ruefully.

Erased the thoughts. Ran a different subject.

The desecration beyond the window will soon be gone.

"Another week, no more, and I'll have your septic buried," the backhoe man assured me on New Year's Eve as he packed up and drove away. "See you in the New Year."

"And us? How much longer before David and I lie covered by this earth?"

My mind wanders before I can stop.

Shivering in the fading light, I run indoors and strike a match. Watch the piñon spring aflame.

As I stretch to pull closed the blind, a swath of pink cloud ices the horizon. Then as it splits apart, reveals the rising orb of a blood orange Super Moon.

I watch its light erode all ugliness — my septic, petty worries of a future that has not yet, and may never happen.

"Come David, How would you like a glass of bubbly?"

It's New Year's Eve. A time of fireworks and Champagne.

We lift our glasses. "Let's celebrate. We've done it darling. Made it through another year."

"Here's to 2018.

63. honest to God...

Last week two well-meaning good friends complained, independently, I might add, that for the first time since beginning my Caregivers' blog over one year ago — a goal I never believed possible — I scored a TROLL.

"You weren't being honest," they accused. I'd avoided what interested them the most... my feelings.

Missing the point, they didn't get it: I was being honest when I wrote I just could not go there... *re-feel* the December the 25th's painful events. Yes, *feel.*

"Enough about David. And the same old, same old," one friend harshly commented. "I wanted your blog to reveal *details* of what so upset you to make the holiday the worst ever. More importantly, what was going on inside YOU?"

You see, dear bloggers and readers, I was in too much agony to face the disaster of that special day so close on the event. Maybe in a year it won't seem so traumatic, and my most un-Christmassy Christmas seem laughable and likely, totally forgotten.

'More of the same... ?' you complain. Well yes. That's how life is for us. One long remorseless struggle attempting to keep hold of what precious elements remain left of the wonderful LIFE that once was ours.

Take my foolish expectation of us sharing an intimate and romantic

Christmas lunch...

Fool. Oh foolish me. Old ways of living can never be.

So I confess, I did cop-out as my friends asserted. Same reason I never fire-walk, bungee-jump or brave the Ropes Course either — A wuss maybe, but by blanketing pain in a whiteout of non-thought., a sort of self-protective mechanism, you might agree, I save my emotional body and avoid hurt.

Same strategy when I was a child and one day found my mother gone. Not able to express my painful thoughts and feelings, I made up the *my-mum-was-stolen-by-a-badman* story in explanation of my mummy's absence.

Though make-believe is dead, and today's villain is the Parkinson's thief who tries to wrench the two of us apart... rob me of my David... my friends have no notion of the building terror raging inside me some days, which, if expressed, might render me useless as a caregiver. Mostly I can button my mouth and prevent some nasty comment from slipping out.

"It's NOT David's fault," I constantly gag myself on the good days.

Not THAT day, though, that Christmas Day, two weeks ago.

"You're killing me," I blurted, clutching at the pain stabbing my shoulder. "My body isn't strong enough to take it any more."

Bedtime. The TV off. I pulled at his body physically unable to get David standing.

"And Parkinson's is killing me," David could have re-joined. Didn't of course. He's way too nice. Just looked crestfallen.

He fell back onto his chair flopped awkwardly leaving the two of us hurting; him, from the indignity of his helplessness; me, from the distress of witnessing his suffering; us from our collective pain.

"There must be a way to solve this. We just can't go on this way," we both weepingly agreed.

Hospice? Ingest a happy pill? Arrange in-care help?

No. No and no.

Solution: Accepting we needed help, next day we called two strong men to move the auto-lift chair from the shed into the living room. A temporary aide to tide us over. All the effort it takes to get David to his feet is a press of a button. Changed our lives.

Who cares if the chair's garish red doesn't match the soft green of our living room. I did, of course, but bit my tongue.

Time to tell it as it is; Parkinson's is a progressive disease. And a damn cruel one at that.

With only one sure outcome, no solution but the end – the D-I-E-word no one speaks of, David and I have come to the peaceable agreement for him to die well. A good lesson for me, I might add.

As David's wife, as his caregiver, my task now is to help him die better. Could be a couple of years, a month or two, or the two weeks David fantasied. No matter the timing, we no longer skirt the subject. After all the process of dying is hardly new.

"My God, your arms and legs feel like blocks of ice," I remarked as I helped him to bed.

"What's going on with your circulation? Or... ?" I recoiled. "Is it the life-force leaving?" I stuttered at the obvious explanation.

"More like it," David assented.

"Oh, my sweetie-pie," I replied for it was stupid to deny its significance.

This week our hope for a return to normal life burned out. Acceptance of David's slow dying has surprised us with an unexpected calm and greater intimacy.

January 20, 2018

64. change of heart

Blog number 5, the *think your home is your castle* one... I vehemently declared my home had been invaded. It's walls breached by a horde of experts till my castle became more like a market place. How I resented our lack of privacy back then. Physiotherapist, Occupational Therapist, Speech therapist, a weekly nurse and who only knew who. Wanted their cheerful faces out of our home.

Was I so stupid to so unwillingly accept their help? Yup. I sure was. Couldn't wait to see the front door close behind them.

That was then. No more.

"Come in. Come in," I barely turn my head nowadays to see who is entering the front door.

8.30 Monday/Wednesday. Ah that must be Kindly-Mr K. He stays an hour and a half to get David up and breakfasted.

Tuesday/Friday. A trumpet call to hounds, *You've gotta get up. You've gotta get up* announces the arrival of the Respite Worker from Senior Services as he blasts David from sleep. I cover my ears gritting my teeth and smile good morning. A jazz trumpet at that morning hour is amusing once. Every visit... ? Hmmn... David and I now used to his ways, humor him.

Thursday. M, our renter-David-helper is the designated person to get David up and ready so I can take him to The Parkinson's Choir Group in town. Till as recently as two months ago it used to be the other way around, me dragging David from bed and rush-rushing to get him ready on time, and M, our renter-David-helper taking David singing. Woke up and got it right at last. Found the better way to look after me.

By the time Saturday and Sunday arrive, I'm ready for *Our Day* — David's and my alone time. I almost like helping David get dressed, and even revel in the breakfasts shared… the scrambling of eggs and spoon-feeding him and buttering toast. Quiet times Just the two of us.

The lessened stress unravels the worry-temper lines on my face. Relaxes my neck and shoulders.

"My, you look better," a friend noticed.

"Yes. I've buckled under and am getting more help," I grimace. "Means gouging into David's hard-earned savings but heck that's what he worked to hard for. I've finally convinced him. The future we've been saving for is NOW."

Trying to think of what constitutes *taking care of yourself,* as people are so glibly advising, I couldn't come up with much. For in truth we caregivers have as limited a choice as an indentured servant who wields no control of her own life — Parkinson's, in my case, being the brutal taskmaster.

Money is the decider, I've decided, the factor that makes possible taking care of yourself. Dollars. Lots of them. $$$$$$$$. Yes, sad to say taking care of one's self costs. Money for a sitter, money for any little help, and as for Respite Care or 24 hour care… well that would break the bank.

Dreams like a day at a Spa… still waiting to experience that particular luxury… would be a treat… having some willing person serve me my evening drink for a change, being told to sit tight while that same imaginary angel fetched it… forget such nonsense.

"Oh to be my own person again," I sigh.

"Any time you want help," friends say concerned, "I'm there for you. Just let us know."

"I'd love that," I sigh again, thanking them knowing I can never take them up on their generous offer.

I erase the improbable thoughts: a social friend wiping David's mouth? Dealing with his toileting or wrestling his dead weight body from his chair and moving him safely? Hardly.

If truth be told, the times when I most need help, most people are still abed a morning, or flopped out after supper cozy before the TV.

Having learned not to kick against what cannot be changed I get through the most part of most days without too much hair-pulling. Though I confess, I do allow a little *Goddamn-it-not-again* cursing to escape my lips when I feel about to explode.

I don't like myself for being such a foul-mouth, but venting is one effective way to take care of myself.

I have found other ways. Simple ways like sneaking breakfast on my own, enjoying the *aahh* first sip of morning coffee before David wakes. Then on the occasional day when I know we'll be home alone and expect no-on to come knocking on the door, I treat my-self to a *no-bra-no-shoes-day* as I call it and dress in my slops.

I've discovered my most pleasurable pleasure — being granted just a little time to meditate and set my intention for the day. Those mornings I can creep from bed and leave David snoring, and breathe in the Champa incense wafting from my puja.

Today's contemplation suggested I consider my ups and downs as no more important than the fluttering ribbons of a maypole, and I, the real me, at the center, firm and enduring as its pole.

Now that reflection refreshed my spirit.

Two days ago David's whistle woke me. Damn. It was 5.30 a.m.. Blast. The clock read one a.m. when I finally fell asleep.

"The only way I'm getting out of bed at this hour is," I growled determining to take care of my own needs for once. "... if you're desperate to use the toilet."

That said we both closed our eyes and slept.

"What ever made you call for me?" I asked more kindly rising sometime after seven, after an extra hour.

"I felt lonely, and wanted you to hop in bed with me," he replied looking sad.

"Oh darling, why didn't you say?" I exclaimed overcome with shame.

If missing such opportunities is what comes of putting myself first... taking care of myself, I've decided, comes well and truly second.

I dread the hour before bed when I have to prepare everything and I dread the getting up in the morning when I have to sort everything. The days run into each other but they are empty days. Only my phone alarm to remind me about medication. I am lucky he enjoys sitting in his chair and reading most of the day. It is hard to go out and walk as he has so much pain walking and my heart is in my mouth until we are safely back in the apartment once more if we do go out. I think to myself, how can we continue this way? ~Carol C.

January 27, 2018

65. the disease that waits for none

My Caregiver Role took an unexpected twist this week. Never saw it coming, but suddenly there I was at the Round House last Wednesday at 8.15 a.m. with a mike in my hand "testifying" to the House Committee how a Movement Disorder Clinic in New Mexico would benefit David's and my personal situation.

Unimaginably there is no such facility, and only two and a half Movement Disorder Specialists in the State. And they are so inundated by the clamorings of the States' Parkinson's sufferers, it takes between nine and eleven months to get an appointment. Follow-ups included.

If it were heart-rending testimonies the Committee wanted to hear, then they got what they asked for — six testimonies to be exact — four Parkinson's sufferers and two Caregivers spilled their stories — better than none at all, but a paltry sample of New Mexico's Parkinson's population, nearly 10,000.

I resolved to be short and not so sweet when my turn came to tell David's story.

To serve a visual punch I flashed a pair of before and after photographs — the first showing David from eighteen months ago frozen lopsided with his eyes closed during one of his catatonic episodes — often lasting perhaps forty minutes at a time — dismissed by local doctors as *normal Parkinson's freezing.*

"Hardly normal," I countered each time to their brush off, before gathering up David and taking him back home.

"Not satisfied with the diagnosis," I continued, "I surfed the web for the nearest Movement Disorder Clinic, clinics adequately equipped to thoroughly test and treat people with movement disorders.

Having set up an appointment, I bundled David into the car and journeyed the long distance out of state to Phoenix, Arizona.

After three days and nights of David wearing an ambulatory EEG and me following with a camera, the specialist discovered David's so-called *normal Parkinson's freezing* was in fact not normal at all but an easily treatable condition.

"I found something," he clapped his hands, delighted. "The left temporal lobe of his brain is continuously seizuring, most likely a reaction to one of his medications."

The specialist smiled. "No wonder he cannot speak, nor open his eyes or move."

"And," I paused, looking at the committee members round the table, "here is my husband now after correct diagnosis and treatment... "

I flashed an upright-sitting-smiling David showing his trans-formative resurrection AFTER the Phoenix Movement Disorder Clinic prescribed a simple seizure med and gave him back his life. Mine too.

The committee took the point:

Sufferers of such a debilitating disease should not be forced to travel out of state to receive the specialized testing and treatment they need.

New Mexico may be one of the poorest states in the country, but isn't the U.S., too, one of the world's wealthiest countries? But that's another issue.

*　　　*　　　*

A PROGRESSIVE DISEASE WAITS FOR NO MAN.

Presented with confusing cocktails of prescribed medications I can't imagine if we had to wait nine months to find and eliminate the culprit medication causing new and scary symptoms... Hallucinations being just one example.— *he'd most likely have either been locked up as nuts, or be dead.*

I still have nightmares when I think back to David's psychotic event — the night he tried to drag me to the car at 3 AM to flee with him from the terrorists about to arrive and burn down our home.

"But if we leave here, the police won't know where to find us and tell us what to do next. What about a spot of tea while we wait." I played along. Coaxing him to stay was an AWFUL experience.

.I feared David's superhuman strength, the wildness in his eyes, and remember the gripping terror... the imminent danger of his driving off into the night, should he spot the car keys enticingly, dangling by the front door. The stress of talking him down with my fingers on the dial button poised to call 911.

David and I are lucky our local neurologist, though not a movement disorder specialist, is at the end of a phone line in an emergency, and sees David every two to three months to monitors his functioning. Has done for 20 years.

*   *   *

The *what if* haunts me. What if we hadn't persisted to get a second opinion about his freezing? I feel sick recalling how hopelessly resigned we felt, and think how unlivable our lives would be today if we'd accepted his freezes as normal.

And what of the vast majority of my Parkinson peers — those thousands of us less fortunate who cannot afford the time or $$$ it takes to keep up the search? I grieve for them.

Thanks to the out of state specialist restoring David's ON times, we're no longer condemned to the isolation of our self-imposed house arrest. The strain of him collapsing in public was just too, too stressful.

I still cringe remembering the cinema crowd held hostage behind us in the auditorium with David blocking the exit unable to move… the restaurants where he's collapsed frozen and once onto the floor alarming the customers…

Oh the glorious difference now he's longer prone to freezing episodes. Confident once more we go to the movies, share a meal out, visit friends.

Along with the five others, I am to testify again this next week, first to the Senate and then to the Legislators from the 'floor' of the Round House.

To both, I plan to end with this plea:

"I ask you all. Please support our Memorial and pass a resolution to provide a Movement Disorder Clinic in New Mexico."

Tonight, let's look back on our lives you and I, because it is obvious they have been interesting and full, and see where we have been and what we have done and close our eyes to what is now and what will be, just for a little while…. cheers! Happy New Year and may 2018 not be too challenging for either you nor I and as peaceful as it can be for D and D. ~Carol!

66. Spoke too Soon

Gathering with so many Parkinson's sufferers and their hard-pressed Caregivers as I did at the Government Roundhouse this past week for the first *Parkinson's Awareness Day* in New Mexico, I came away quite chipper and buoyed by the knowledge David seemed almost athletic compared to some, and I, a spoiled complainer after hearing other Caregivers' stories.

I was particularly moved by the tale of a frail friend of ours who has to hump her severely disabled husband from wheelchair to toilet to bed entirely alone.

Broke, their house under foreclosure, unable to afford $$$ it costs to pay for respite care, the two of them are trapped — he unable to communicate with speech, and she in desperate need of help for her companion.

My friend, like those with partners too disabled to attend the event, bore instead, a photograph of her beloved in her arms — a photo of the *partner-who-was* BEFORE Parkinson's stripped him of all he had been, and cruelly ripped their happy relationship. Smiling, her partner's eyes shone vibrant — and hers from remembering.

So heartbreaking… the photographs… the faces of men and women, young and old as they used be. Alive. Healthy. Living.

David and I *have it good* I am convinced. Well, comparatively speaking that is, I qualify.

I watched a man half David's age cross the hall in front of me... his legs caving, his balance up-ended, he clutched his Care-partner's arm to keep from falling. He — so young and so afflicted, my heart crumpled in empathy, horribly aware some of the battles waiting ahead. David and I being older have so much less to lose. After all, bent though he is, he is still has the physical ability to walk. Has lucid, near normal moments during which we actually converse.

Behind the Caregivers' happy faces, put on for public display, I saw desperation, pleas for help, a cries for comfort. Mirrors of mine?

Am I a soothsayer? No, not me. I say this because in them I see my pain, the sadness of watching our partner's disintegration, the flares of anger, then guilt we feel. Like them, I am entrapped in a life of Caregiving never bargained for when the words I DO were spoken, promising to love in sickness and in health.

I come over so bright and cheerful sometimes, people are fooled I assume, or do they see my grieving, the hollow behind my eyes?

Keeping a lid on it is my British way of coping with emotion you must understand. The only way I am able to keep on going. And going... and going.

Scary things, pressure cookers; I've always been scared to use one... the sight of all that steam escaping... the fear of impending explosion should the lid be unloosened.

Well it happened.

Down in Albuquerque an hour plus from home, key in the ignition, classic music playing, I left David in the car while I shopped. In no hurry for once, I mulled over the unusual selection of foreign groceries fingering, smelling things like Jackfruit, Kuri leaves, snake gourds, and exotic spices, before returning to the car.

"Sorry I took so long, darling," I said pulling to open the door.

It didn't yield. Locked.

"David, David," I called banging on the window. "Open the door."

No response. David sat tilted to one side. The ignition off. Keys dangling.

Banging on the window to get his attention, I began yelling for him to open up. His hand moved, searching, but he was unable to sit up and reach.

"The button... push it... the door handle, pull. Pull."

To no avail, David's fingers crept along the dashboard nowhere close.

Panic. Desperation rising, I looked around for help.

"He's got Parkinson's," I wailed. "He doesn't understand how to unlock the door."

Help came in the form of a woman no more than in her late twenties.

"I'll stay with him," she said. "While you go inside and find help."

The AAA machine phone response crooned I'd won a cruise. I slammed the phone and dashed back outside to check on David. His cheeks glowed red from the trapped heat. Another stranger, tapping on the window to keep his attention, was trying to probe a wire through and trip the lock, but there found no gap.

The young woman pressed her face against the glass calling encouraging directions for David to move his hands up down forward and back. Half an hour had lapsed.

Then just as we were dialing 911, he did it. CLICK. By chance, his fingers stumbled onto the button and the door unlocked.

"Well done David. Well done." The woman said.

Then turning, gave me a hug. "It must be so hard," she comforted. "I'm so sorry."

The kindness of her words undid me. Took the lid off the anguish I keep screwed down behind a smile. And I sobbed. And sobbed. And couldn't stop.

A stream of kind strangers insisted on loading my shopping from the cart to the car. Another gave me a hug and told me to take care… to take a minute… to drive carefully.

David said nothing, made no comment. But, as we drove away, he reached for my hand on the steering wheel and stroked it.

All the 60 miles home, I cried.

I find myself crying again just by re-running this incident.

Yes, it is hard. So hard… the life of a caregiver.

From the outside, no one can judge the level of our suffering.

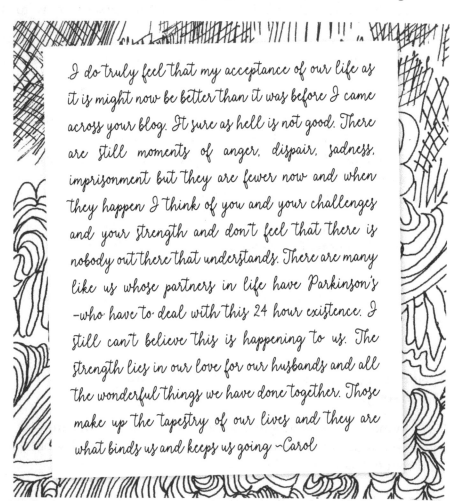

I do truly feel that my acceptance of our life as it is might now be better than it was before I came across your blog. It sure as hell is not good. There are still moments of anger, dispair, sadness, imprisonment but they are fewer now and when they happen I think of you and your challenges and your strength and don't feel that there is nobody out there that understands. There are many like us whose partners in life have Parkinson's —who have to deal with this 24 hour existence. I still can't believe this is happening to us. The strength lies in our love for our husbands and all the wonderful things we have done together. Those make up the tapestry of our lives and they are what binds us and keeps us going ~Carol

February 10, 2018

67. 20:20 i wish
the if only bug has struck.

Used to seeing through a glass darkly for the past few years, the day after my cataract surgery last week, I stared amazed at a world I'd long forgotten. Beautiful. Each blade of grass, cactus thorn, and glittering leaf of the Russian Olive in the garden, and indentation of the rock ridge rising beyond our boundary fence-wire clear in minutest detail.

Living with Parkinson's is like that I realize—a darkening cloud that keeps us veiled from our pre-Parkinson's Disease 20:20 world.

I, David too of course, we've both of us forgotten how easy the most simple activity used to be. We decided to go some place, we jumped into the car and went. Needed a pee? Just a minute's delay. Like a walk? Boots laced on, and away we'd stride through knee-high grasses to climb and sit together on a high rocky outcrop. Can't do uneven ground anymore.

But it's not the same—having to drive a paved mountain road just to gain a view.

I miss the 20:20 experience no longer possible in our world…the exhilaration of treading the iris meadows edging Hamilton Mesa, lying face up to the bluest sky cresting a line of snow-capped peaks in the Pecos Wilderness…the harsh song of Mountain Blue Jay…the sweet burst of wild strawberry.

Since a child I've loved the wild. Remember times when I ran free.

Yes, the *if only* syndrome has brought me down. *If only* David was healthy and Parkinson's hadn't struck… *if only* he could be my husband again and be towards one another as we used to be.

Not all the time, not every day, but these past evenings and mealtimes, such a crest of aloneness floods the house I am swamped lifeless. Slumped flat on the sofa, a cushion under my knees, I've no energy or interest in calling a friend, read the daily news, or pick up a book. I don't care to open or answer my emails. Guess that's how it feels to be…dare I say…depressed?

Sad. Just an immense sadness. That's what I feel. What if people… family, friends, strangers even, caught me like this, happy mask slipped. Empty. And David slumped silent, would they get it, know then, see for themselves the toll PD costs? Perhaps even jolt them into actually do something, find some way to help.

Caregiving weighs too heavy today. I hurt from so much bending. I force myself to stand, pull him to his feet. We head towards the bathroom. Me walking backwards. Guiding. David, eyes closed pulling back.

Life's hard right now. Getting more so. "How ever can we keep going like this? Not good for you, not good for me," I cry. "Me snappy all the time being so exhausted. This is ruining our marriage."

I felt worse when he didn't disagree. Looked at me bitterly.

Hopeless thoughts like these serve only to make me feel worse. Like John Bunyan's pilgrim, keep me wallowing in a slough of despond. Still, if only Parkinson's were like an eye cataract to be incised and tossed away.

Alright, I know I should be used to every darn PD's hardship by now, but actually I'm not. So don't bother reprimanding me for being so negative and ordering me to listen to my own advice. Accept what you can't change.

I know that Okay? Okay. I know my mood will pass. Can't I feel in the dumps just once in a while?

Tomorrow is another day. Better, hopefully. One in which our world spins again in orbit. A day in which we regain our normal happiness.

I clamber into bed. Close my eyes. Reach for a far memory. A glorious 20:20 day of my childhood.

*   *   *

DISCOVERY

my fingers gently part the green   expose wild
strawberries clustered beside a Kashmiri snow-fed
brook   surprise my tongue with their sweetness

in those same woods of rhododendron and pine poke
tiny trefoils   wood sorrel nestled at their mossy feet
I nibble one between my front teeth tasting lemon

above the tree-line below the snow stands a
solitary birch   pale parchment shredding from
its trunk for a raven to scribe his story

deeper between closed forest firs   lurid red and
white spotted toadstools promise eternal rest
lure me to take a bite   but I am not tempted

I step into a knee-high carpet of gentians beside
a snowdrift pitted with imprints where a yeti
passed last winter on his quest towards the sun

*   *   *

February 17, 2018

68. ring-a-ring-a-roses

Well here we both are, David and I merrily dancing one minute, falling down the next. And I don't mean physically, though that happens only too frequently to David and those suffering from the dreaded Parkinson's Disease. I don't know if David quite thinks of our lives as a dance, but I certainly do.

Ring-a-ring-a roses, a pocket full of posies, Atishoo, atishoo, we all fall down... goes the nursery Rhyme.

I never quite understood the meaning of the game I played as a child, but joined happily in the fun regardless, half wanting it to last forever, half not wanting. Oh, the terrifying tension of anticipation, I remember — my fear of falling down mid pirouette just as I was getting into it.

Back during the Black Death, when *Ring-a-Ring-a Roses* first appeared in England, sneezing, I gather, was a first sign a person had fallen victim to the dreaded plague.

Sort of like now.

Merrily, merrily round and round we go dancing life's circle, then boom, a symptom strikes and knocks us for six.

What forces us to us get up over and over again and continue, is one of life's mysteries.

Just like that, one moment here with me in the world, the next disappeared into his private cloud.

Take yesterday. David's sharp quizzing, behaving like any husband would whose wife had not once, but twice, I'm ashamed to confess, turned up at the airport on the wrong day.

"Let's double check if you've got things straight... the correct travel date in June? Flight time? Connections? Confirmed seats? Insurance... All set?"

Today, quite the reverse, David is out of it... a complete goner. Like a sleepwalker, he's spoken not a single word, opened his eyes or shown any awareness I am there helping him to function. Then, come midday up he pops again chatty as can be.

I'm pleased he's back of course, but it's hard for me to switch and take up our dance where we left off.

On to off, off to on. He's here. He's not.

In an instant. No control. No rhyme or reason. David flows from conscious to unconscious leaving me teetering on one foot, so to speak.

True, it's the *same-old, same-old,* I hear you mutter, bored. But what you don't quite get perhaps, is I am taken by surprise every, every single time.

It's the unpredictability of not being able to rely on David's functional presence that so disturbs me.

Each morning I go to wake him wondering who he'll be that day... if he's the David who can, or cannot, lift a cup to his lips by himself... stand from sitting on his own... understand the words I'm saying.

Not that I've ever wanted, or would ever want, our lives to be boring... the *slippers-before-the-fire* and *cocoa-sipping* kind of deadly living, oh no, I love the exciting challenge of variety, the unexpected. I'm talking only of the pleasant, not the traumatic, tragic kind.

I suppose it is wicked of me to have such a thought... my half wanting, half dreading to know an end date to my caregiver role. Likewise life on cruise control.

A young cousin of mine with two teenage boys, diagnosed with a return of her cancer, composed and fulfilled many of the to-dos on her bucket list between her immunotherapy treatments. With her family, she celebrated her twentieth wedding anniversary on a tour of the Kluane Ice-fields; floated, free-falling from the sky; plunged the blue waters of Australia's Barrier Reef scuba diving... on and on she danced life to the final step fully aware of her impending end.

I opened and read her goodbye letter.

"I have less than six months left to live." Her words blurred on the page.

My brave, and lovely cousin, I'm sad to lose you.

I sort of envied her knowing. Sufferer. Caregiver: David. Me. Would knowing our timeline make life easier and bring some comfort, I wondered.

I like to think we would be goaded by the knowledge to follow her example... and to actually do some of the to-dos of our bucket list.

Fulfill David's personal wishes for example. Our joint dreams too, as couple. We've talked tentatively of spending a second honeymoon together somewhere exotic. But to turn dreams to reality? That's the puzzle. Perhaps we'll revisit the Santander beachside hotel where we'd had such a fun weekend when *the rain in Spain* poured relentlessly.

"Hey, David, how'd you like to take a side trip there while we're in France this summer with our family?"

"I like it," he looked up and smiled.

February 24, 2018

69. ZZZZZ... i wish

I heard him fall asleep an hour ago. Heard, I say, because as I cozied down beneath my comforter in my own bedroom across the hallway, staccato snores spat arrhythmically from David's monitor keeping me awake. I should be used to the noise by now, I'd have thought — the apnea-like stops and starts of his breathing.

I pop into his bed sometimes but never make it through the whole night. The wild flailing of his arms and sudden violence of his kicks put my life in peril.

No exaggeration. Fellow Parkinson's Care-partners relate similar dangers and how they too were forced to flee the marital bed. One Care-partner I know related her husband's sleep-thrashing left her with a bruised cheek and near broken nose.

Wakeful, the snorts emitting from the monitor remind me of the years we slept together in the same bed.

Before Parkinson's struck, and David was suffering from sleep apnea when it was all the rage, a concerned therapist persuaded David to hire one of those C-pap contraptions after a fitful night spent in a Sleep Center. Against my better judgment, I might add.

"Is it worth it?" I moan. "What with the discomfort of sleeping with something stuffed up your nose, its infernal trailing tubes, and labored wheezing?"

David barely slept a wink.

"Nor me," I add when he told me.

"If you believe in destiny or fate, David, and accept the premise that we're granted a specific lifespan, then you should trust the machine won't add one day more," I snapped after three turbulent months of disturbed sleep. "Think about it... you're still alive and kicking after years of what's nowadays known as apnea symptoms."

Proving the point with a little tickle, he let out a squeak. That did it. We took the risk, and sent the marriage breaker packing.

The C-pap gone, David slid gratefully into dreamland. Though his breath still stopped mid-exhale as frequently, and was as scary as ever, whenever his next shuddering intake was too long in coming, I'd just dig him in the ribs as I'd done for years and jumpstart him.

Back in the present, I begin to worry how I'll function come morning. List the jobs I know will weigh heavy. Know my temper will be short. I'll have no patience. The night before I slept a miserly three and a half hours, the night before that, just four.

Count the night hours left available... long to fall into slumber... If only I knew how to let go of consciousness.

Sleep deprivation is par for the Caregiver's course, I suppose.

Come 9 PM, just as the descent of tiredness prepares me for day's sweet end, the physical effort of getting David ready and tucked up into bed rewinds my natural body clock from off to full on, till by the time David is all tucked in and my head hits the pillow, *pouffe*... all chance to slip into the land of nod — gone.

Lying there alone, I watch a twinkling satellite speed across the sky, my mind struggling to unravel the morning's contemplation.

"Sever all bondage. Abandon your old dwelling."

I focus on the enigmatic message, and drift asleep.

March 3, 2018

70. abandon your old dwelling

I mulled over this morning's contemplation.

Is it time then to stop writing this weekly blog? I'm feeling *blogged out* you see, emptied of any more to say. About Caregiving, that is, not writing in general.

Words I have thousands of… piling up like one giant snowdrift, which if I don't *pen* soon, threaten to melt away.

Lying in my room alone in bed, staring into the night, struggling to unravel the morning's contemplation, I watch a winking satellite slice the sky.

SEVER ALL BONDAGE. ABANDON YOUR OLD DWELLING.

I focus on the enigmatic message. Scan the words for a deeper meaning. Come up with this garbled interpretation.

In this world, the world binds you… but you *CAN break free* by re-inventing yourself…

CAN BREAK FREE, now there's an idea I can go for.

Yes, perhaps I'm being told it's time to move on. Not from David. Not from looking after him, for like the subject of Robert Frost's famous quote, *I have miles to go before I sleep* but to move on from a *Care-giver* to being David's *Care-partner*. For recently I've felt a change come over me; the budding of new hope.

Talk about a slow learning curve to get the lesson:

David. + Me. + EFFORT = PARTNERSHIP.

When I first became my David's Caregiver I felt life reinvented me, and stole my right to carve my own path in this world. Frightened, angry, and in pain for us both, I lost my way toppled by David's escalating symptoms.

Wishing myself free, I'm being held against my will, has been my constant moan since then. Can it be at last, that today I'm over with wishing? Wishing circumstances different than they are. Wishing myself the perfect Care-partner I'm not. Most of all wishing David's crippling disease away. And his full health and vibrant self back.

I talk to myself a lot to pass the hours before I sleep.

"Accept reality, fool." I scolded one such night last week. "… no point in useless wishing."

I punched my pillow in emphasis. "All too easy to say, but how, how, how?" I argued with myself, grumbling inwardly, scanning the night-sky for inspiration.

My mind wandered to Rani, an Indian girlfriend of mine. To her story. Married off to a stranger against her will in an arranged union, I remember her explaining how she came to accept and ultimately love the man she found herself bound to.

I couldn't resign myself to being owned by somebody, so after a hellish couple of years resenting my entrapment. Then, like a train switched to a different track, I mentally took back my power and chose to serve him. At the same time, made the choice to wholeheartedly adopt my new country. The minute I made up my mind, the only things I could change were my own thoughts and behavior, I began to almost love the man. Now we adore each other.

She smiled, I remember.

If only I could change and think like Rani. Take back my own life, and in the process, happily co-exist with my new owner — you know, that damnable Parkinson's thief. I can't weep forever.

Note: I said co-exist, not LOVE.

There is no, nor ever will be, some imaginary fairy descending from the sky with her magic wand to disappear our uninvited guest.

Nope. Parkinson's is here to stay. Goes without saying sharing our lives with it is abnormal — dreadful, and cruel if truth be told.

Imagine at my advanced age having to drag a grown man from room to room with his eyes tight shut, struggling to manhandle the weight of him to his feet, feeding, walking, talking is just not normal.

Certainly not the golden years I planned.

"I'm not born to this," I've too often yelled. Still do sometimes. "I just can't do it any more."

Running on overdrive as I do, I've learned to excuse my occasional crankiness and vented steam as no more than a disguise to hope-less grief of loss.

"It's only natural," friends console when I confess, ashamed.

It just happened. That one particular night in bed alone last week. In the midst of all my mental chatterings, I felt an avalanche of love. I felt suddenly euphoric. I simply loved the man. No matter the disease's relentless batterings, we would weather this.

Suddenly scared of losing a single moment together, and that our precious time could soon be gone, I scurry now from my bed to his room, breath in the living warmth of him, sneak my hand across his belly and sleep.

"I've been nicer," David overheard me telling a friend.

"It's true. You have. I can feel it," David looked up at me and smiled.

Re-reading my first blog of over a year ago, Wearing a Hat from Hell, I see I've changed, so I am getting ready to wrap up my blog.

Today, this week, this month... who knows if I'll have any words to add. And if I don't post regularly, please understand and let me know if you want to keep in touch.

Dear unseen bloggers, I thank you all for your support in responding so generously. I have learned so much both from and in talking to you.

*   *   *

Our story has no neat progression as found in a novel. No *ah-ha* moment, no epiphany, or neat arc to round off the manuscript as an author might. No, David's and my lives are one long series of rollercoastering symptoms flinging us from despair to hope in never-ending loops. So many reversals — ups and downs — we barely have strength enough to make it over the next hurdle.

We are planning where David would like to spend our second honeymoon.

No dark tunnel for us. David's dying journey, our journey, will be in the open and most beautiful countryside we can imagine.

Our own story, the book still to be completed, lies open waiting for its pages to be filled. Unfinished. It glares no longer blank.

Scribed by the two of us together, some entries will bring pain. Some memories of unimaginable joy.

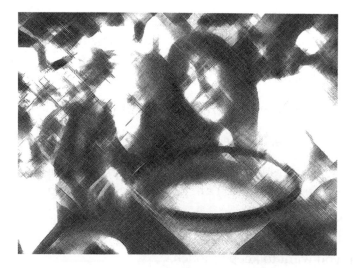

appendix

TAKE CARE OF YOURSELF, indeed. How? Any suggestions?

How about an allowance USA to pay the dollar cost of residential inpatient care costs we've saved you? And I might be able to pay for a little RNR time to myself. An oil massage would be nice...an hour or two shopping un-burdened by my PD partner...mmm...a meal on my own with a friend... oh to spend a few days alone.

Struggling to lift David's legs onto his bed, I dream of winning the lottery, a windfall, a donation from some generous charitable organization willing to pay for an aide to lighten my load, the kindness of some undercover boss or philanthropic person with the financial power to ease David's and my lives.

Let's face it, reality is respite help is a fantasy most of us cannot afford. I and all caregivers of PD partners and other incapacitating disabilities, will slave till exhaustion kills one of us or both.

In the meantime here is a list that may help:

COMPASSION AND CHOICES— www.guidestar.org/
end of life option act, medical aid in dying.
End-of-Life Options (EOLO) Coalition

BEING MORTAL— Dr. Atul Gwande's book on-
maintaining autonomy as we age

MEDICATION OPTIONS— took a lot of trial and error over years before discovering David was more alert and functioned better on less rather than more. Neurologists took a lot of convincing that the tiny amount of medication he was taking could be of any benefit until they saw him in action.

EXERCISE. EXERCISE. EXERCISE—David loves Walking, singing and treading the treadmill. Hand:eye:brain co-ordination such as Rock Steady Boxing, a Chair Strengthening Class.
Ping Pong is our favorite sport—something he can succeed and beat me at—The difference in David's balance and focus is unbelievably improved..
Think Loud And Big: Physical therapy created for Parkinson's sufferers. We use their method to keep David striding out instead of shuffling. No longer a stick or walker for him unless he asks.
https://www.lsvtglobal.com/clinicians
LSVT's DVD for home practice. + check out YouTube videos from Ohio demonstrating the reduced time it took an elderly PD sufferer to put on his jacket and to get up and down off a chair.
Easy Yoga for Arthritis video—Peggy Cappy.
Really got David moving. And safely.

GAME-PLAYING—not to win but to stimulate mental skills, bearing in mind both auditory comprehension, verbal expression, visual perception and memory. No need to list which games, just play any activity that takes your fancy....Rub-i-cub, Suduko, Dominoes, Poker, Scrabble, Set, Word Search. Who cares how simple, simple works.

BOOKS FOR THE BLIND—Free to those who like David cannot keep his head still enough to read, nor his fingers nimble enough to turn a page or click a Kindle

PARKINSON'S TRIALS —check eligibilty to be included. w.w.w.clinicaltrials.gov

MOVEMENT DISORDER SPECIALIST AND CLINIC—head for the nearest location as soon as your Parkinson's partner has been diagnosed. For us unequivocally worth the expense and travel to keep treatment on track, and without whose deeper diagnosis and care I doubt David would be functioning as well as he does. Here's-a-pill-and-see-you-in-a-year doctors just don't cut it for us.

WEBINARS—bound to be a mine of valuable info but as yet no time or computer brain to try one out.

LOCAL SUPPORT, COALITION AND ACTION GROUPS—
wish now we'd braved our New Mexico Advocacy group years
ago. Monthly meetings with specialist lectures, demonstrations,
and a yearly conference, through them we've discovered in-valu-
able information as well as made new and supportive friends.

SENIOR CENTERS—free classes, meals, free transportation
and social contacts. Ditto to the above.... We delayed going
for way too long. Matt, our amazing chef welcomes us both
by name. Saves caregiver-me food shopping, cooking and
washing up. Another plus—interesting silver hairs and baldy
attendees to chat with over a meal, plus friendly staff.

SENIOR SERVICES—free if you and your Parkinson's
partner qualify. Our Respite Worker gets David up and
shaved and fed. Gives me two hours off a week.

CAREGIVERS GROUPS —such as info@caregiveraction.org

INSPIRING VIDEOS—
—"Blame It On The Parkinson's" song/video by Mitch Faile. A
song so poignant I both laughed and cried.
—Neuro Film Festival from the American Brain foundation www.NeuroFilmFestival.com "One Day With
Parkinson: 9-6-13" Tom Seawell's film of Mark's personal experience living with Parkinson's says it all.

PARKINSON"S ORGANIZATIONS—
—Davis Phinney Foundation for Parkinson's—
www.davisphinneyfoundation.org
Look for the Victory Counts Manual
—Michael J Fox Foundation—www.michaeljfox.org
—APDA American Parkinson's Disease Association
www.apdaparkinson.org
—Muhammad Ali Center in Phoenix, AZ
—Brian Grant Foundation—briangrant.org
Brian's inspiring story of summiting Mt. St. Helens
with PD renewed my determination.

CPSIA information can be obtained
at www.ICGtesting.com
Printed in the USA
FSHW02n1707070618
49064FS

9 780986 118869